Incorporating Science, Body, and Yoga in Nutrition-Based Eating Disorder Treatment and Recovery

I0131137

Incorporating Science, Body, and Yoga in Nutrition-Based Eating Disorder Treatment and Recovery is a valuable, innovative guide that demonstrates how clients and clinicians can untangle, discern, and learn from the complex world of eating disorders. With voices from every stage of recovery, this book illustrates how clients can claim mastery in food and life. As a nutritionist who specializes in disordered eating, the holistic method Ms. Mora created provides individuals with a true potential for healing.

Incorporating Science, Body, and Yoga in Nutrition-Based Eating Disorder Treatment and Recovery weaves strong, resilient, and vibrant threads of science, dietetic .practice, and yoga therapy that harmonize with all treatment modalities. It will help treatment providers from every discipline to guide clients as they reweave their lives with nourishing relationships, embodiment, and ongoing growth.

Maria Sorbara Mora, MS, RD, CEDRD, CDN, PRYT, RYT, is a registered dietitian and yoga therapist. She is Founder of Integrated Eating Dietetics-Nutrition, PLLC in New York City, Brooklyn, and Garden City, NY. She's treated people with eating disorders since 1999.

Joe Kelly is a best-selling author, editor, educator, father, and grandfather in Richmond, California. Formerly a Minnesota Public Radio regional news director, he co-founded the international, award-winning, girl-edited magazine *New Moon Girls* and the national advocacy nonprofit Dads and Daughters. Kelly helps health and education professionals to mobilize and utilize their clients' and students' male loved ones as resources and coaches men with family members suffering from eating disorders and/or addiction.

Incorporating Science, Body, and Yoga in Nutrition-Based Eating Disorder Treatment and Recovery

The Integrated Eating Approach

Maria Sorbara Mora and Joe Kelly

Routledge
Taylor & Francis Group

NEW YORK AND LONDON

First published 2020
by Routledge
52 Vanderbilt Avenue, New York, NY 10017

and by Routledge
2 Park Square, Milton Park, Abingdon, Oxon, OX14 4RN

Routledge is an imprint of the Taylor & Francis Group, an informa business

© 2020 Taylor & Francis

Library of Congress Cataloging-in-Publication Data
A catalog record for this title has been requested

ISBN: 978-1-138-58429-7 (hbk)
ISBN: 978-1-138-58430-3 (pbk)
ISBN: 978-0-429-50610-9 (ebk)

Typeset in Bembo
by Swales & Willis, Exeter, Devon, UK

To my two children and husband. I love you with all my body, mind, and soul. Maria

To Dr. Margo Maine, trailblazer, mentor, and friend. Joe

Contents

Acknowledgments

Both of us thank Routledge, Amanda Devine, Sonnie Wills, and Daradi Patar for bringing this book to you. We especially thank the wonderful Carolyn Costin who "introduced" us while Carolyn and Joe created the book *Yoga and Eating Disorders: Ancient Healing for Modern Illness* (Routledge, 2016). Many thanks to the energies and inventors who created pathways for us to write a book together across 2,919 miles.

From Maria
Conceptualizing, writing, and rewriting this book is a process of evolution and integration.

Divine intervention is truly to thank for the kick in the soul to get this book out to the world. Therefore, my first and foremost thanks is to the Source.

To my loving husband: Thank you for supporting me on this writing journey and for putting up with countless hours I was missing in action and for the anxious moments in between. For tending to the kids, supplying me with endless coffee, kombucha, and kisses and for your spirited energy. During the final stages of writing, I overheard you on the phone speaking to someone and saying, "My wife is writing a book on nutrition for eating disorders. She's wanted to do this since we met." Well, 13 years later, it has materialized. You are my anchor.

To my beautiful children: Thank you for your enthusiasm and for making room for my laptop on our kitchen table, on your desks, and basically anywhere else in the house I could put it. This book literally and metaphorically brought another seat at the table.

To my daughter: You are wise beyond your years. You asked if there was a place for the "life cycles" in this book. The answer is yes. Right here. Like a caterpillar becoming a butterfly, the people in this book undergo a metamorphosis of body, mind, and soul. I am honored to work with them.

To my son: You remind me often of what is important in this world, so you are one of my most influential teachers. I appreciate your patience with me and my process. I look forward to bedtimes and snuggle time without my computer in tow.

Thank you both for inviting me on bike rides to the park with Dad now that "you are done with your book." I am a very lucky mommy.

To my parents, siblings, grandparents, and other family members: Of all the riches you supplied in my life, the joy of family meals is among the most dear. Growing up in our old-school Italian family meant grandmothers making fresh pasta, pizza, and cookies, while grandfathers bottle tomato sauce. My mother Carmela (one of the world's best cooks) never makes the same recipe twice, but always puts in the most important ingredient: love. My father Marino grows his own chili peppers and lettuce. He moved our fig tree with us from Brooklyn to Long Island. I learned organic farming before it was cool. In short, food *is* family. When we are together, sharing food is a sacred and blessed act of connection. Thank you for this most important lesson in feeding. While we all talk with our hands, we feed from our hearts.

Yogic traditions call us to give gratitude to all those in the seen and unseen realms who walked beside us on our path. Ancestors and angels, teachers and mentors. I thank:

- Richard Shear for his continued "school of life" support
- Mary Segerra, my career mother figure who took in a young clinician and provided supervision (and so much more) in the specialty of eating disorders
- Phoenix Rising Yoga Therapy, especially my teachers Elyssa Cobb and beloved Karen Hasskarl, Michael Lee, and Soleil Hepner for training me in the most important pose: witnessing with positive regard.

To those who have invoked the divine feminine here on earth: Katie Dove Hendon, Dechen Rheault, and Marilyn Genoa.

To Carol Hoenig for preparing my proposal and doing the groundwork for this book's publication.

To Carolyn Costin: You are my inspiring role model. Early in my practice, a client went to California on scholarship to receive treatment from you and your team. She told me you were a healer. A true trailblazer in holistic recovery, you inspire in me a genuine desire to heal with heart and from the heart. I was so honored to write for and receive your most valuable feedback while contributing to *Yoga and Eating Disorders*. I am grateful that book led to co-authoring this book with Joe. What a gift. Thank you.

To Joe Kelly: While working with you on my *Yoga and Eating Disorders* chapter several years ago, I remember feeling amazed by your special gift for making words come to life. Working with you on an entire book was a dream come true. From the bloopers and blunders created by talk-to-text to the late-night edit calls, you gave me a lifetime lesson that one's voice on paper is a sacred gift. Thank you, thank you, thank you.

This book is a tribute to my past and present patients and their incredible recovery journeys. I am blessed to have you as wonderful teachers. You remind me that we are all here to grow, change, heal, conquer our greatest fears, and emerge true warriors. Accompanying you is a privilege that I do not take lightly. Please know each and every one of you provide me with precious life lessons.

From Joe

Many thanks to Dr. Margo Maine and Rev. Dr. Steve Emmett for welcoming me into the community of people working with those affected by eating disorders and advocating for eating disorders care. I also thank the following dear folks who taught and still teach me about eating disorders and community: Carolyn Costin, Dr. Pamela Carlton, Stephanie Brooks, Signe Darpinian, Katie Bell, Michelle Minero, Dr. Anita Johnston, Clayton Uyehara, Bridget Whitlow, Katherine Westin, Dr. Matthew Kaler, Dr. Lisa Rogers, Lisa Diers, Stacy Sainden, Michael Kieschnick, and especially Heather Henderson.

For showing me how much fun books are to write, I'm thrilled to have decades of gratitude for Robin Dellabough and Rosalie Maggio. Many thanks also to one of the world's most supportive friends, Bob Stien.

My family provided wonderful support during the book's composition. Big hugs and love to my children Nia Kelly, Mark Stelzner, Mavis Gruver, and Jon Sung and my grandchildren Sam and Quentin.

Working with Maria Sorbara Mora is a treat and an honor. During our first joint venture back in 2015, she opened my eyes to many profound similarities between writing and yoga. Those insights continue giving breath to my sentences. Thank you for inviting me to work with you again. I admire you!

Enormous gratitude to my more than marvelous spouse, Nancy Gruver.

We thank Ellyn Satter for permission to quote from her book. *Secrets of Feeding a Healthy Family: How to Eat, How to Raise Good Eaters, How to Cook* (Madison, WI: Kelcy Press, 2008).

Introduction

Invisible threads are the strongest ties.

—Friedrich Nietzsche

To be effective, eating disorders treatment and recovery must address multiple, complex layers of the person's life: body, brain, bones, other organs, intimate relationships, family, reproduction, spirituality, emotions, psychology, career, friendships, finances, and more. To be effective, treatment must, at minimum, provide medical, psychological, and nutritional support from eating disorders-trained professionals. Not surprisingly, treatment and recovery have multiple, complex layers and usually take substantial amounts of time.

No matter why or how someone embarks on their recovery journey, they'll regularly confront an existential question: "Who am I without my eating disorder?" Early in recovery, this seven-word question may feel impossible to answer; or the answers may seem uselessly ephemeral. Nevertheless, clinicians and clients must ponder this question seriously, because it captures:

- the enormous leap of faith clients must make
- the terror of stepping away from familiar eating disorder ways, and risking eating disorder retribution
- the terror of stepping away from familiar eating disorder ways and being overwhelmed by life
- the terror of stepping toward the as-yet-unknowable path of recovery.

Despite the terror, people can and do recover from eating disorders. However, they don't do recovery to become "normal" eaters. Recovering from the depth and breadth of their eating disorder experience demands learning how to nourish body, mind, spirit, and relationships with self and others. Recovery calls people in our care to accept imperfection, while practicing gratitude for all it teaches. Recovery calls them to practice joy, hope, faith, service, and ease-full mastery in eating—and life.

This book gives an overview of a detailed, interconnected, science-, dietetic-, and yoga-based process. If you are not an eating disorder-trained Registered Dietitian or yoga therapist, we strongly suggest working with one to implement Integrated Eating in your practice.

If you're not familiar with eating disorders, you need to separate facts from myths before going any further.

Eating disorders are real, complex, chronic, and serious illnesses. The American Psychiatric Association's *Diagnostic and Statistical Manual* recognizes binge eating disorder (the most prevalent eating disorder), bulimia nervosa, anorexia nervosa, other specified feeding or eating disorder (OSFED), and avoidant restrictive food intake disorder (ARFID).

All eating disorders lead to malnutrition. Eating disorders last anywhere from months to decades. They are dangerous, life-threatening, and under-diagnosed. Most people with eating disorders never seek or receive treatment. Eating disorders are usually accompanied by other health problems, including (but not limited to) addiction, posttraumatic stress disorder (PTSD), anxiety, depression, obsessive-compulsive disorder, type 2 diabetes, organ damage, tooth erosion, osteoporosis, attention deficit hyperactivity disorder (ADHD), personality disorders, and sleep disorders.

Eating disorders are not choices or fads, any more than cancer or type 1 diabetes are. People from every ethnic, socio-economic or geographic background develop eating disorders. So can people of any gender and any stage of life, including childhood. Like with cancer, we don't know exactly what causes every eating disorder, although there's consensus that biological, psychologic, genetic, and cultural influences are factors.

People with active eating disorders, and people fully recovered from them, describe the illness as an abusive partner, a narcissistic sociopath, a life raft, a seducer, a protector, a part of the self, an enemy, a lover, a teacher, and an existential threat. Here's another image:

> It was like a monster was living inside of me, telling me how to act, what to eat, and how to feel about my body and my life.

They are baffling, clever, devious, disruptive, hard to discern, irrational, powerful, secretive, stubborn, unfair, and unjust. Eating disorders hijack the sufferer and their loved ones. There are some things that we and the disorder can never understand about each other.

Bottom line: eating disorders are overwhelming and draining to live with. Hence, they often are overwhelming and draining to recover from.

Integrated Eating

Integrated Eating is a four-phase process that incorporates the body, mind, and soul to support eating disorder healing and recovery. It guides patients as they learn mastery over symptoms, mastery in self-nourishment, and mastery in living. Patients may leave and return to treatment for various reasons during or after any phase—most often because they are, or are not, ready for the next step.

Phase 1: Structured Eating

Basic structures of eating go out the window in an eating disorder. Chaotic eating blurs the lines between eating events, distorts portion perceptions, and leaves the body in danger. Our patients must relearn how to eat. During Structured Eating, we share the science of macronutrients and how they meet the body's changing needs throughout the day. Patients schedule six or seven balanced eating events a day (breakfast, lunch, dinner, a mini-meal, and floating snacks). They learn layered skills, like how much food to consume at each eating event—and how to prepare or obtain it. They practice meeting the body's changing needs by eating *prescribed* food in *every* eating event. The Structured Eating phase takes frequent nutritional support and sustained, repetitive practice of elementary skills.

Phase 2: Mindful Eating

Once the people in our care master Structured Eating skills, we add the layer of mindfulness. Patients learn how to use their senses and sensations to collect information about their eating and food experiences. Mindful noticing-without-judgement is difficult for brains and bodies ingrained with eating disorders' judgment-first, sense-distorted mindset. However, sustained Mindful Eating practice will deepen a patient's connection to eating and body.

Phase 3: Intuitive Eating

Here, patients use information they gather through mindfulness to practice discerning, choosing, and taking action. Sustained conscious practice creates neural pathways and body memory that clear away eating disorder debris obstructing communication with inner wisdom. Wisdom already exists, layered in the person's being. For example, before the brain can consciously discern the body's current need for omega fatty acids, a healthy body will crave fish. In Intuitive Eating, patients practice unblocking and trusting their inner wisdom's speed-of-light discerning, choosing, and acting processes (otherwise known as intuition). Intuitive Eating is a huge leap forward for patients, and usually demands more practice than the first two phases.

Phase 4: Mastered Eating

This "final" phase is a life-long practice that seeps into every layer and thread of the recovered person's life. Mastered Eating is not perfect eating. Fortunately, our world and our lives are gloriously and naturally imperfect.

The client's countless days of practicing form, mindfulness, and trusting inner wisdom create transformation. Mastered eaters continue to integrate their skills and practices in the service of continual learning, responsibility, compassion, trust, joy, gratitude, and service to self and others. They cherish how imperfection provides room to give and receive connection and grace. They know that our souls rely on fresh air coming through the doors and windows of our imperfections.

Every Master Starts at Love Point

What characteristics come to mind when you think of Serena Williams? Profession: tennis player. Champion (highest-ranked player in the world on eight separate occasions between 2002 and 2017). Olympic gold medalist. Strong and resilient (reaching the Wimbledon finals nine months after giving birth by cesarean section and suffering a pulmonary embolism). She embodies what it means to be an elite player, even though she still loses games, sets, and matches.

However, we'd never describe her as someone who *simply* plays tennis. Athletes like Williams dominate tennis, define tennis, become tennis. They are masters of tennis. But how do they earn this title?

Once upon a time, future masters knew nothing about tennis. They have no wins or points. So, how do they weave their way to mastery? The very first thread was learning what tennis is, at a very young age. They watch older players hold a stick attached to a circle with tautly woven strings. They observe the older players hit fuzzy balls back and forth across a low net. The child doesn't fully understand what the players are doing or why they're doing it. Even scorekeeping is cryptic: zero points is called love, one point is 15, two points are 30, three points are 40, and five points are game (if you win by two points).

The next thread is learning the most elementary form of tennis. Novices must identify a racquet and layer on the skill of holding it. They learn where to place their feet. Then they must learn how to swing the racquet in ways that hit the tennis ball. Then, they must practice resilience and fortitude to handle rarely getting the ball over the net. Learning these rudimentary tennis skills requires repetitive, structured practice.

Eventually, growing proficiency helps the determined player make mental, physical, and emotional connections among the layers of sensations, movements, and outcomes. For instance, they notice that swinging the racquet too hard makes the ball go out of bounds. Use too little force, and they see how and why the ball can't quite get over the net. They become mindful of how body and mind affect their particular play: hand grips, balance, movement, and swinging style. They rarely get past love point, but their skills have more ease. They still practice.

With years of practice, patience, and determination, a player like Williams becomes an elite competitor. With help from her parents and experienced coaches, she discerns and integrates her preferred grip, stances, and swings. She discerns frustration with losing and euphoria with winning—and chooses what to do next. Informed by that information, she develops layers of strategy to make best use of her strengths and compensate for her weaknesses. She learns to be at the right place at the right time to make the next shot.

Over time, Williams seems to understand (before her conscious brain knows) where the opponent will aim the ball. Her body, mind, and spirit move to make the next shot, while anticipating the opponent's *next* volley and her *next* response shot. She's practicing a deeper layer of knowing: intuition. Of course, intuition alone doesn't score points. Williams still must do her best to hit the ball where she intends to, while understanding that her best doesn't guarantee winning the point, or any other outcome. She still loses games, sets, and matches. Determined to get even better, she keeps practicing ... a lot.

Then, mastery happens. Something changes, but it is difficult to articulate precisely. Williams seems to be everywhere a split second *before* the right time. The tennis novice turned experienced professional turned mastered player walks on the court "in the zone" and soars. She seamlessly comes back from 40–love to win a game. And it happens again, and again. From championship to championship.

The transformation is palpable and not fully describable. The integrated layers of structure, mindfulness, and intuition catapult the person into the realm of tennis artist ... tennis genius ... tennis master.

Integrated Eating's Threads

Integrated Eating's goal is healing. We support a person with an eating disorder to practice basic, structured eating; learn mindful eating skills; become an intuitive eater and ultimately experience mastery (not perfection) in life.

We developed Integrated Eating by weaving strong, resilient, and vibrant threads of science, dietetic practice, and yoga therapy.

Successful healing from an eating disorder requires more than just untangling its complex warp and woof of behaviors and consequences. Successful healing means weaving or reweaving life with relationships, embodiment, and ongoing growth.

Registered Dietitians utilize Integrated Eating to collaborate with other providers. We support healing and recovery by guiding clients to discern and learn from eating patterns and relationships. Those skills transfer seamlessly to the rest of a client's recovery and life.

To be clear: we are not (and don't pretend to be) psychological therapists. We are nutritionists who understand eating disorders, treatment, and recovery. We support treatment and recovery with applied physiology, nutritional science, dietetic practice, yoga therapy, and client experience.

Integrated Eating is organized and fluid, scientific and yogic, uncomfortable and nourishing, difficult and often fun. Developed in an outpatient setting, it incorporates learning and language from multiple disciplines. Clinicians and clients use the knowledge and lingo to discuss, motivate, and integrate the multiple facets of treatment and recovery. Integrated Eating is a nutrition treatment modality which:

- serves a patient's nutritional needs
- serves the rest of a patient's treatment team (therapist, physician, etc.)
- reinforces the work and goals of a patient and their treatment team

Rooted in rigorous disciplines and years of treatment experience, Integrated Eating uses:

- evidence-based and eating disorder-attuned nutrition support
- applied physiology
- patient education in nutrition, digestion, metabolism, and neuroscience
- yoga-informed nutrition support
- eating disorder-attuned yoga practice
- trauma-informed yoga practice
- yoga and nutrition embodiment.

The Thread of Science

As we detail in later chapters, eating disorders manifest and rely on distortion, denial, myths, and mistaken beliefs. Transparent and explicit use of scientific evidence is a powerful therapeutic treatment tool. (A quick note: we use "therapeutic" in its broadest definition; nutrition, psychotherapy, medical care, spirituality, yoga, somatic work, spiritual practice, and creative arts are all therapeutic.)

Throughout every phase of Integrated Eating, we talk with patients about the relevance and science of nutrition, applied physiology, anatomy, biochemistry, microbiology, human biology, urology, endocrinology, neuroscience, organic and inorganic chemistry, kinesiology, research, and replicable experimentation. As this client acknowledged, the information helps—and takes a while to sink in:

> My dietitian and I had many emotional discussions about my not keeping up my end of the deal by not gaining weight. I learned the science of what would happen to my body if I didn't consume fat. After about a year of treatment, I finally reached my goal weight.

Here are some things explicit science education accomplishes for patients and clinicians:

- It provides scientific methods and verifiable research to validate what happens when clients encounter, perceive, and/or misperceive their lived experience.
- It establishes solid, scientifically verifiable foundations and rationales for therapeutic interventions.
- It scientifically explains steps of the recovery process.
- It demonstrates that multiple treatment and recovery skills are equally critical, and how they link, interact, and propel recovery.
- It dispels myths, challenges denial, and disarms treatment skeptics.
- It creates form and format for translating science and science education into digestible parts that patients and clinicians from all disciplines use in sessions (e.g., over-exercise activates the sympathetic nervous system, which then exacerbates restriction, anxiety, and additional sympathetic nervous system activation).

The Thread of Dietetic Practice

Professional dietitians are trained in nutrition science: the study of food, and food's relationship to the human body. When we eat food, our bodies digest, absorb, and utilize macronutrients, vitamins, and minerals to meet the body's diverse needs.

Because I am a Registered Dietitian, people sometimes ask me: "What does the average dietitian do all day?" I usually start my reply by saying: "There is no average dietitian." Registered Dietitians provide renal nutrition, cardiac nutrition, oncology nutrition, pediatric nutrition, holistic nutrition, weight loss nutrition, pregnancy nutrition, sports nutrition, endocrinologic nutrition, nutrition for people in poverty, hospice nutrition, diabetic nutrition, hospital nutrition, and nutrition education. Some of us provide eating disorders nutrition.

The common thread is feeding for wellbeing. Food is the vehicle, eating is the road, and the destination is health and wellbeing.

In eating disorder treatment, dietitians are first responders using food and eating to stabilize people with severely malnourished and unbalanced bodies. A patient may arrive with blood sugar instability, dysregulated metabolism, blunted fullness/hunger cues, malfunctioning organs, inability to manage medications, and/or compromised mental function. As my patient Ellen says:

> In the beginning of my sophomore year of high school, at the age of 15, I often sat in my classes feeling productive because I was thinking solely about the number of calories I'd already consumed that day. Consuming fewer calories would help achieve my goal of perfection, to be thin. Little did I know I was battling with a horrible disease.

Clear, candid nutrition education, structure, and direction facilitate feeding and provide other benefits to patients and clinicians:

- nourished patient body
- bridges to understanding why nutritionists ask patients to do specific things
- connection to palpable patient sensations, behaviors, and consequences (e.g., hunger/fullness, eating balanced foods, shift in energy)
- experiencing nutrition "education" in real time ("You told me that if I did *x*, then *y* would happen. It was different when I saw it and felt it myself")
- strengthened connection and communication with the body
- reminders that the client has a body
- reminders that the body relates and responds to food
- openings to heal relationship with body, mind, and soul.

In eating disorder treatment, dietetic practice is indispensable. Talk therapy is very difficult when the patient's body and brain are malnourished. We can't treat someone who dies of malnutrition-induced heart failure.

Eating disorder dietetics isn't for the faint of heart. Because lives depend on it, Registered Dietitians must be tough, direct, and honest.

The Thread of Yoga

Yoga practice and yoga therapy are common modalities for eating disorder treatment, with good reason. Neuroscience research is showing yoga to have positive impacts on depression, anxiety, addiction, PTSD, and eating disorders. Embodiment lives in the DNA of both recovery and yoga.

Ahimsa, yoga's first ethical tenet or *yama*, means non-violence. The disruptions of eating disorders (e.g., dissociation and blunted sensations) violate the body, mind, and soul. Treatment disrupts that harm by challenging clients to inhabit their physical body more fully through the process of feeding. This means patients must metaphorically bump up to their material body's edges—a necessary *and* painful experience.

Integrated Eating grew from Mindful Based Stress Reduction (MBSR) and Phoenix Rising Yoga Therapy to provide clients with safe spaces for exploring physical sensations, thoughts, and emotions. When practicing structure, awareness, and discernment, clients become present to the realities of their body, mind, and soul. They develop deep trust in the body's guidance.

I can hear a clinician or two thinking: "Whoa there, my friend. Where are you going with all this soul stuff? I can't get on board with that sort of thing."

Like you, I value skepticism. Early in Integrated Eating, we teach patients the scientific method (aka, systemized skepticism) and its utility as a recovery tool. The shared experience and practices of psychotherapists, Integrated Eating dietitians, and yoga therapists reveal mutual resonance. They reveal significant overlap between established mental health concepts and yogic conceptions of soul and inner wisdom.

- dialectical behavioral therapy (DBT): wise mind
- Freudian psychology: ego
- acceptance commitment therapy (ACT): valued direction
- internal family systems (IFS): the self
- cognitive behavioral therapy (CBT): accurate information
- dietetics: inner eater
- eye movement desensitization and reprocessing (EMDR): cognitive insight
- 12-step programs: conscious contact
- gestalt: whole forms

In real life, most eating disorder treatment providers come to see yoga, nutrition, psychiatry, talk therapies, and somatic therapies as synergistic partners. Each modality stirs up *and* contains therapeutically necessary experiences. Yoga helps patients embody the challenge of exploring their edges *and* experiencing safety in their body. We can also practice yoga in nearly any setting. Partnership between modalities provides amazing, integrated, and mutual support for healing.

Eating disorders (and their common comorbidities) are traumatic life events. When we experience trauma, our body stores the impact on a deep cellular level in muscles, fascia, joints, organs, nervous system, and the brain. As trauma researcher Bessel van der Kolk, MD, says: "The body keeps the score." The body responds to this profound somatic integration with physical ailments, mind distortion, emotional instability, and spiritual unrest.

Yoga therapy helps to process and heal what trauma leaves behind by leaning into parts of the body where trauma is stored. It uses breath, movement, mindfulness, meditation, and the grounded pillars of yoga philosophy.

Yoga therapy and yoga practice do numerous things for people with eating disorders:

- increase body responsiveness
- aid body acceptance
- reduce disordered eating thoughts and tendencies
- decrease cortisol
- facilitate compassion
- strengthen parasympathetic nervous system response
- strengthen recovery intentions
- reframe "disorder" energy as creative energy.

Yoga therapy and yoga practice also provide clinicians from different disciplines additional language to use when treating patients and collaborating with other members of the treatment team.

Where We're Headed

Each Integrated Eating phase develops patient intention. Integrated Eating practitioners have intention, too. We intend a practical, comprehensible, and effective process for the people in our care. Here's how one of those people described her experience:

> Early on, I was just so thankful that we were looking at my eating disorder and my body in a concrete, conceptual way (if that doesn't sound contradictory). I still fought back, but (at the same time) I "got" the science behind how, for example, my eating anxiety fires up my sympathetic nervous system and creates this crazy, endless loop.
>
> I didn't hear anyone say I was doing something *wrong*. The calm, matter-of-fact conversations about the science of my body opened up a way for me to see (or begin to see) the reality inside my body. The door opened slowly, but just enough to trust (most of the time) the plan for what needs to happen first, what needs to happen next, what needs to happen after that, and who needs to be involved with it.
>
> Even when the eating disorder was in full chaos mode, part of me felt that I was getting guided through the scaffolding of my potential recovery. I was learning how to build on it. Looking back, I can see that I wasn't alone with my eating disorder; I had the treatment team, the science, the food, the yoga practice, and my body.

Recovery means looking honestly at the parts of life which are overloaded and/or fried by an eating disorder's highly charged power. It means looking honestly at where in life eating disorder patterns may still cloak themselves. This hard work is worthwhile because recovery short-circuits the energy of an eating disorder, and its influence on the person's life. It frees the people in our care to be who they are without the eating disorder or its energy. Plus, recovery's transformation seeps blessedly into other parts of life.

Yoga philosophy considers intention as a sacred, focused, and creative energy that manifests in transcendence. That's a familiar concept to most mental health professionals. As clinicians, we are in the field of recovery to live our purpose and guide our patients towards their potential and purpose. The journey is long, but not linear. It asks clients and clinicians to look deep within to find what yoga calls "our lotus in the mud," the lesson in the story.

Please note:

1. We share vignettes about and conversations with clients throughout the book. To respect and protect their anonymity, we changed their

names and many identifying details. We feel deep gratitude for their wisdom and feel honored to share it with you.

2. Because people of all genders have eating disorders, we use the inclusive word "they" as a singular *and* plural pronoun. We occasionally use "she" and "he" within stories about clients who specifically identify as female or male. If you're unfamiliar with the singular they, we ask you to be patient; you will probably get the hang of it.

3. This book has two authors but is written in the voice of Maria Sorbara Mora.

Bibliography

American Psychiatric Association. *Diagnostic and Statistical Manual of Mental Disorders*, 5th Edition (Arlington, VA: American Psychiatric Association, 2013). 307.1–307.50

van der Kolk, B. *The Body Keeps the Score: Brain, Mind, and Body in the Healing of Trauma* (New York: Viking Penguin, 2014).

Yehuda, R., Daskalakis, N.P., Bierer, L.M., Bader, H.N., Klengel, T., Holsboer, F., and Binder, E.B. (2016). Holocaust exposure induced intergenerational effects on FKBP5 methylation. *Biological Psychiatry*, 80(5), 372–380.

Youssef, N.A., Lockwood, L., Su, S., Hao, G., and Rutten, B. (2018). The Effects of trauma, with or without PTSD, on the transgenerational DNA methylation alterations in human offsprings. *Brain Sciences*, 8(5), 83.

1 The Person, the Disorder, and Recovery

Eating disorders dis-order our instinctive, inborn human relationships with food, eating, self, and others by (in effect) making them all about numerical values (calories, weight, steps, miles, amounts of time I spend with so-and-so, etc.) and formulas (when and where to binge, purge, restrict, excess-ercize, deny reality, avoid so-and-so, etc.).

As a result, clients are in pain, even if they don't yet fully realize it. When people step through our doors, for the first or the forty-first time, their walking is talking. By showing up, they are saying: "I need help!"

Of course, our clients have been in pain for a long time already. Pain is a concrete and vibrant "I need help!" message from the body, mind, and/ or spirit. For months, years, or decades, an eating disorder responded to the call for help. Its "answers" are rigid, narrow, and formulaic:

- Obsess over every calorie, fat gram, etc.
- Obsess over eating or not eating.
- Learn and practice how to purge with the least discomfort.
- Binge every time you feel discomfort or uncertainty.
- Purge every time you feel discomfort or uncertainty.
- Restrict every time you feel discomfort or uncertainty.

The eating disorder and its answers are ultimately unhelpful, harmful, and dangerous. They do not heal, but they do serve a function. They *temporarily* provide:

- sensation numbing
- release of sensation-stimulated tension
- sensation denial
- distance from reality and self
- predictability
- armor against appearance-based harassment and objectification
- distraction from sensations, reality, self, others, and life.

Unfortunately, all of these "answers" distance the person from their body, its pain, and healing. None of them lead the client closer to whatever is generating the pain and its message.

None of them answer (or even ask) the question: "What part or parts of me *need* help?"

By the Numbers

Obsession with weight is a common eating disorder pattern. It also runs throughout the complex constellation of body image, body awareness, body acceptance, body satisfaction, body distortion, and underlying self-worth.

All of these problems blur and/or deny a simple fact: weight is a number calculated by a math and physics formula (more on this in a bit).

When patients compulsively try to "control" their weight, obsess about weight, hate their appearance, and/or are dismissive of their body, clinicians must recognize:

- This *obsession* is information.
- This information signals that the client is entering the black hole of body image.
- Our job is helping patients recognize and explore the pain represented by that black hole.
- We can't effectively do that by arguing about the physics formula $w = mg$.

What is $w = mg$? Newtonian physics defines an object's *weight* (w) as the value of how the *mass* (m) of that object is influenced by the force of *gravity* (g). To measure something's weight, multiply its mass by the acceleration of gravity. At this moment, in the universe, acceleration of gravity varies dramatically by location. At this moment, my mass is constant.

Scientists measure *mass* in kilograms and weight in Newtons (Isaac gets so many perks). On earth, every object with a mass of 1 kg weighs 9.81 Newtons.

Life outside the laboratory is more confusing. At Target, the "kg" number on a laundry detergent box refers to the contents' weight, not its mass. Depending on local custom, we weigh our produce in kilograms or pounds. The British measure weight in "stones" and call their currency "pounds." As if physics wasn't hard enough already! As the scientists say, "I don't buy potatoes by the Newton, but I do research by the Newton." Junior high science detour ends here. Deep breath!

Say your weight on earth is 100 pounds. Your body's mass is 45.3592 kilograms. If you travel to the moon this afternoon, your body's mass will remain 45.3592 kilograms, but the acceleration of gravity is just 16.66 percent of gravity on earth. Therefore, you'll *weigh* a little over 16 pounds on the moon. If you visit the International Space Station (ISS), your weight will be zero. That's what weightless means: without weight (*not* without a body).

Imagine stepping on a scale on the moon. Now imagine doing it here on earth. Both scales calculate the same thing: our body's mass times the acceleration of gravity. (Sorry, no can do on the ISS; you need gravity to stand on a scale.)

Weightless ISS astronauts and cosmonauts still have relationships with their bodies. You and I have a relationship with our bodies, no matter where or whether we calculate our mass times the acceleration of gravity.

Eating disorders and body image problems live in *that relationship*, not in *numerical values* like weight, gravity, mass, calories, pounds, stones, ounces, feet, meters, or inches.

Humans have relationships with all manner of people, places, and things (including gravity). As my co-author's daughter once said while maneuvering a piece of furniture: "Remember, gravity is our friend!" It sure helps when moving furniture down the stairs. It's very stubborn when moving furniture up the stairs.

Clinicians must understand that, when clients obsess about mass times the acceleration of gravity, they are communicating information about their:

- relationships with food and eating
- relationship with their body
- relationship with their authentic self
- relationships with other people, places, and things.

As clinicians we must resist one-dimensional responses to "$w = mg$" obsessions. Instead, we read between the metaphorical lines to help patients journey away from "I am my weight" beliefs, practices, and neural pathways. Effective treatment gives people consistent, "non-$w = mg$" eating and body experiences in the practice of self-care, self-acceptance, and self-love.

Of course, treatment and recovery don't remove *mass times the acceleration of gravity* from the world. But they do offer the potential for transformed relationships with people, places, and things (like gravity). As a recovered friend puts it:

> I now see weight for what it really is: one bit of data (among many, many others) that *may, at times,* provide *some* (but not all) useful information about how I am caring for my body. I rarely think about weight any more, which is quite liberating.

The barriers to healing and transformation are massive. And they are frequently occurring opportunities for us to guide and support our patients to put weight in its proper place at the proper time: one bit of data about mass and gravity. We usually need to focus on this data point early in recovery, and occasionally later on. Otherwise, we put $w = mg$ on the shelf with other data, like the dictionary.

It Ain't the Numbers; It's the Relationships

Throughout Integrated Eating, we remind our patients: "In recovery, your body must come first. Despite what an eating disorder says, feeding your body and feeling its presence are more important and useful than using symptoms to (temporarily) numb and/or disconnect from your body."

For example, we ask the people in our care to imagine a small child approaching an adult:

> The child, too young to get her own meals, asks the adult: "Can you give me something to eat?"
>
> In a sharp tone of voice, the adult immediately answers: "Not now, I'm busy."
>
> After a few minutes, the hungry child begins crying and pleading for food. The adult grows more agitated and impatiently replies: "No! I have important things to do."
>
> The crying continues and (if the adult bothers to look), they see a child in pain. This enrages the adult even more. They shout or growl: "Go away and leave me alone!"

We talk with the patient about the story and their reaction. We ask how they feel about the adult. We ask how they, in real life, would treat this hungry child (or any hungry child).

They say: "Well, I'd never treat them like that! That's crazy. That's cruel. Who would do such a thing? I would never deny a child food when they're hungry." We notice, acknowledge, and name their compassion.

Next, we suggest: "Imagine your *body* is a small, hungry child." We often see jaws drop as patients perceive the parallels between:

1.   the heartless adult and their eating disorder
2.   the hungry child and their body.

Finally, we ask them to consider treating their own body with the same compassion they give a hungry child. We ask them to practice saying this to their body: "Yes, I'll put down what I'm doing. Sit down, child, so I can feed you now."

The hungry child story illustrates a disordered and distorted human relationship and its consequences. I believe that obsession with $w = mg$—in eating disorders *and* in our culture—is symptomatic of a disordered and distorted perspective on the function of human relationships.

When people with eating disorders get "stuck" on calories and $w = mg$, I suggest that the eating disorder places far more value on calories and weight than a miser does on money. Then I ask: "Are rich, miserly people the only people worth having relationships with?"

Healthy and fulfilling relationships between people aren't determined by numerical values or formulas. Relationships don't have mass controlled by the acceleration of gravity. Human relationships are created and developed through the interactions and responses of the two (or more) parties involved. Any "weight" or "gravity" we assign to relationships is purely metaphorical.

Each of us has a relationship with food and eating created and developed through the interactions and responses of the eater and eating. Living, breathing, and genuine relationships are scary for people seeking safety in the rigid, formulaic (and false) certainty of eating disorders.

In short: it ain't the numbers; it's the *relationship*.

Eating disorder treatment and recovery happen in and through relationships. Treatment and recovery pivot on the person noticing, accepting, and growing in their relationship with food, eating, people, places, and things. Recovery has other major benefits, because it usually expands a person's capacity to accept, value, and grow in relationships with other people, spirituality, community, career, and so forth.

Inspired by influential therapist and dietitian Ellyn Satter, MS, RD, LCSW, BCD, we created a chart of characteristics to help illustrate the point (Table 1.1). The first two columns (on the left) compare disordered eating with Ellyn Satter's characteristics of normal eating.

The second two columns (on the right) compare disordered (e.g., abusive, codependent, etc.) human relationships and fulfilling human relationships between people.

Please note: the Normal Eating column is Ellyn's work, which she graciously permitted us to use. Everything else in this chart is our own interpretation.

Take a few moments to reflect on the comparison.

Did you notice that the "Disordered" columns have more repetition than the other two columns? Did you notice how (and why) the "Natural" and "Fulfilling" columns convey more variety, flexibility, and trust?

Table 1.1 illustrates the many ways that eating disorders make a person's perspective and experience narrow, rigid, self-harming, and harming to others.

To help move patients "from the numbers to the relationship," eating disorders treatment providers use a variety of medical, psychotherapeutic, and nutritional modalities.

Relationship with Self

Integrated Eating makes regular use of yoga practice and yoga therapy. We find yoga helps patients learn to explore and contain the self–and their relationship with the self.

Table 1.1 Eating and Human Relationships

Disordered Eating	Normal Eating	Disordered Human Relationships	Fulfilling Human Relationships
Obsessively and rigidly bingeing, restricting, etc.	Is eating competence. It is going to the table hungry and eating until satisfied	Hide and deny needs for emotional, relational, spiritual (etc.) connection	Feed your natural human hungers for connection, meaning, comfort, etc.
Compulsively restricting, bingeing, purging	Is being able to choose food you enjoy and to eat it and truly get enough of it; not just stop eating because you think you should	Avoid new or different people; maintaining contact with very few people	Do not end just because someone or something else disapproves
Compulsively exercising, restricting, bingeing, purging	Is being able to give some thought to your food selection so you get nutritious food, but not so wary or restrictive that you miss out on enjoyable food	End for fear of difficult emotions, other people's opinions, cultural constructs	Dedicate thought and intention while inviting and deepening your relationship, so you are nourished spiritually, emotionally, psychologically, etc.
Fear-filled "rules" about food (indulge, deny, restrict, purify, cleanse, etc.)	Is giving yourself permissions to eat because you are happy, sad, or bored, or just because it feels good	Hide and deny needs for emotional, relational, spiritual (etc.) connection. Try to control the other person's behavior	Give yourself permission to be together with another person sometimes because you are happy, sad, bored, or just because it feels good
Fear-filled "rules" about food (indulge, deny, restrict, purify, cleanse, etc.)	Is mostly eating three meals a day, or four or five, or it can be choosing to munch along the way	Judgmental, rigid, and fear-filled "rules" about other people and relationships	Inviting and being involved with people and situations that are truly and mutually fulfilling
Compulsively exercising, restricting, bingeing, purging	Is leaving cookies on the plate because you will let yourself have cookies again tomorrow, or eating more now because they taste so great!	Blame others for how you feel. Try to control the other person's behavior	Can mean being together occasionally, regularly, and/or nearly all the time

(Continued)

Table 1.1 (Cont.)

Disordered Eating	Normal Eating	Disordered Human Relationships	Fulfilling Human Relationships
Fear-filled "rules" about food (indulge, deny, restrict, purify, cleanse, etc.)	Is overeating at times, and feeling stuffed and uncomfortable, and undereating at times, and wishing you had more	Feel abandoned by others. Resent and try to control the other person's behavior	Can survive "overload," recognizing the need for autonomy and occasional time away from one another. Can survive separation, recognizing how absence makes the heart grow fonder
Bingeing and/or purging to self-punish for "mistakes"	Is trusting your body to make up for your mistakes in eating	Feel smothered by others. Resent and try to control the other person's behavior	Enjoying and embracing people and situations different from what you are used to
Thoughts, attention, and energy overwhelmed by food/eating obsession	Takes up some of your time and attention, but keeps its place as only one important area of your life	Feel abandoned by others. Resent and try to control the other person's behavior	Take time and attention, but is not the only important area of your life
Compulsively exercising, restricting, bingeing, purging to avoid difficult emotions	In short, normal eating is flexible; it varies in response to your hunger, your schedule, your food, and your feelings	Hide and deny thoughts and feelings. Try to control the other person's behavior	Develops instincts and intuition; trusting your emotions, sensations, and wisdom, etc.

Yoga grows from non-Western, contemplative, and spiritual perspectives of reality. Yogic philosophy perceives five subtle sheaths or layers of self, known as *koshas.*

Think of an onion's layers. Each one has characteristics; some are like other layers and others are different. All the layers connect to one another. "Separately" and together, all the layers are infused with onion-ness. They all manifest onion-ness. No two onions are exactly the same, but they all have layers. And they are all onions.

Yoga philosophy views humans as beings with layers. Each person's layers have characteristics; some are like other layers and others are different. All the layers connect to one another. "Separately" and together, all the layers are infused with human-ness. No two people are exactly alike, but we all have layers. And we are all human beings.

The five *koshas* or layers/sheaths:

- influence one another, like one pebble creates ripples throughout a pond
- are interconnected
- manifest the self
- shape the self's stuck-ness
- shape the self's growth and transformation.

Annamaya is the sheath of our material body, considered the densest layer of our being. The material body needs balanced nutrition to survive and be well. For people with eating disorders, the most immediate distress and strife reside in the *annamaya* layer. Experienced treatment providers know that feeding the material body appropriately will keep it alive and reduce its distress and strife. Integrated Eating spends time with, treats, and begins to heal *annamaya kosha* in Structured Eating. *I eat foods that align with my meal plan.*

Pranamaya is the sheath of life force pulsating through every part of our being. Our breath and senses manifest our vital energy and bring life force to the self. Eating disorders stifle vital life force energy through deprivation and malnutrition which unbalance and stress our body. During Mindful Eating, we practice connecting to *pranamaya* layer by using our senses to bring awareness to our experiences. We continue to nurture *pranamaya kosha* with yoga, meditation, and breathing practice. *I use my senses to engage with food. I sense my body experience before, during, and after eating. I am grounded and embodied while I eat.*

Manomaya is the layer of cognition and emotion. Our mental and emotional consciousness inhabit this deeper layer of self. Eating disorders harm *manomaya kosha* through thought distortion, emotional numbness, emotional instability, anxiety, and depression.

We develop our mental and emotional consciousness through mindful and intuitive eating practices. *I notice relationship patterns between my body, eating, thoughts, and emotions.*

Vijnanamaya kosha refers to the wisdom and new knowledge we draw from our unique being and higher mind. It includes discernment and will. Eating disorders create mounds of spiritual and emotional debris that weigh down the sheath of wisdom and block our access to *vijnanamaya*. Through the Intuitive Eating phase, we practice discerning patterns, learning from them, choosing the next right thing, and doing the next right thing. The practice helps us gather innate guidance from deeper parts that have been waiting patiently to be tapped. We seek out our body's wisdom and listen to all it has to say in all our relationships. We learn to trust our gut, heart, and mind to intuit what we know deep within the self. *I listen and consult with my body about its nutritional, relational, and spiritual needs.*

Anandamaya kosha houses our Atman or True Self. Yoga also calls this sheath the "bliss body." In Mastered Eating, we practice allowing the wisdom of *vijnanamaya kosha* to penetrate and direct our lives. We practice finding zones of "flow" where we discover new knowledge, insights, perspectives, healing, and growth. As recovered or recovering people, we can embrace acceptance, compassion, and forgiveness. We no longer regret the eating disorder or other past pain; now we see each experience as *one* of our many spiritual teachers. Eating and food become joyful and full of human connections. We realize that our True Self has joy, empathy, resilience, trust, hope, and the urge to be of service. All the gifts and grace are available when we are ready to tap into our authentic, true self. *I connect with my food, my body, and others in joyful eating and life experiences.*

A Sacred Sandwich

Throughout Integrated Eating, we strive to see eating as sacred communion with self and other people, places and things. Think of the mundane peanut butter and jelly sandwich (PB&J): all it embodies, all it represents, and all those who created it.

Take a few moments to meditate on gratitude for the community of things and people (including you) with whom you join before, during, and after you eat a PB&J:

1. wheat kernels, sugar beets, soybean plants, peanut plants, and fruit vines, trees, or bushes
2. the sun, air, rain, soil, and planet
3. every person who plowed, planted, tended, and harvested each ingredient
4. every person who builds and maintains machinery that helps plow, plant, tend, harvest, and transport each ingredient
5. every person in the factories that use each ingredient to create bread, peanut butter, and jelly
6. every person who packages and transports the bread, peanut butter, and jelly

7. every person who unloads the bread, peanut butter, and jelly, stocks it on the shelves, and/or collects the money you paid for them
8. every person in the factories that built the grocery store shelves, scanners, cash registers, carts, and signs
9. every person that built the grocery store
10. the person who made your PB&J: you, a family member, people in a factory that supplies sandwiches to your 7–11
11. the people you're eating with (including you)
12. your five senses
13. your digestive system
14. the protein, fat, complex carbohydrates, fruits, legumes, vitamins, and minerals in your PB&J
15. the ways your body converts the entire sandwich to meet its needs
16. the ways your sandwich provides energy and helps to rejuvenate your muscles, become your cell lining and bolster your organ tissue—all so your body can serve you.

Some people with eating disorders come out of this meditation with shame: "OMG, all those people got involved in my life, and I failed them all." In recovery, the people in our care learn to practice letting go of shame. By counting themselves as part of larger communities, their embodied belonging nurtures liberation from the eating disorder.

Yoga provides distinctive and practical ways for clients to choose nourishment over deprivation, curiosity in lieu of judgment, mindful awareness instead of numbing, and appreciation over denial.

Sustained yoga practice (like practicing gratitude for every participant in a meal's journey to your table) facilitates eating disorder recovery. It brings the possibility and promise of connection that transcends the disorder and everyday life experience.

After all, a PB&J is far from mundane. Food unites the earth, growth, body, self, and other people. Eating unites nutrition for our survival with nutrition for our relationships.

Besides tending to the sacred inner eater, we connect with the soul by cultivating an authentic relationship with ourself.

Recovery is a long, non-linear journey calling people to find and connect with their innate inner wisdom; their guiding source. Recovery never calls people to be perfect. It asks us to nourish, honor, and listen to our mistakes, progress, practice, and life force. Recovery calls us to continue practicing and progressing toward deeper connection to self, others, and beyond.

Bibliography

Costin, C. and Kelly, J. (Eds.) *Yoga and Eating Disorders: Ancient Healing for Modern Illness* (New York: Routledge, 2016).

Georgia State University Department of Astronomy. *Mass, Weight, Density.* http://hyperphysics.phy-astr.gsu.edu/hbase/mass.html. (Retrieved April 13, 2019).

Roeser, R.W. An introduction to Hindu India's contemplative psychological perspectives on motivation, self, and development. In M.L. Maehr and S. Karabenick (Eds.), *Advances in Motivation and Achievement, Volume 14: Religion and Motivation* (Amsterdam, NL: Elsevier, 2005). pp. 297–345.

Satter, E. *Secrets of Feeding a Healthy Family: How to Eat, How to Raise Good Eaters, How to Cook* (Madison, WI: Kelcy Press, 2008).

2 Structured Eating Foundations

Eating disorders—no matter what form they take—result in a disordered relationship to food *and* a nutrient-distressed body. Therefore, the first order of recovery business is to feed the body what it needs. After all, it's extraordinarily difficult to attempt psychotherapy with someone whose brain is malnourished and not functioning well!

Integrated Eating begins with Structured Eating, which trains (or in some cases retrains) the body to effectively communicate its nutrition needs to the brain, so that body and brain work together in the eating process. It is the crucial first phase for a patient getting treatment.

In acute levels of inpatient care, the nutrition/feeding model is usually three meals and three snacks a day, because the patient's malnutrition must be addressed immediately (remember that all eating disorders—including binge eating disorder—create malnutrition).

An Overview

Structured Eating is a concrete process which trains the body and brain to synchronize. Structured eating gives organization to food and feeding through nourishing balanced meals, mini-meals and snacks throughout the day.

Structured Eating begins mechanically and continues repetitively; that is, the patient routinely eats meals and snacks built to stabilize the body's feeding and metabolism functions by using:

1. a clearly defined eating pattern
2. clearly defined intervals between meals and snacks
3. a balanced and effective way of eating.

When people walk through our doors, they often feel out of control. We created Integrated Eating's first phase to honor this reality. We don't find it wise to overburden early-treatment patients with too many things. The Structured Eating phase is extremely concrete. It focuses intently on the concrete process of *what to do next.* "Eat within the first hour after waking up. Eat every three or four hours until you go to sleep. Here's your meal and snack plan." That's a lot for new patients to handle in their first five or six sessions with us.

A dietitian must set the meal plan parameters during the Structured Eating phase, because the eating disorder and nutritional imbalance (resulting from the disordered eating) arrest the patient's ability to plan restorative feeding. At the beginning, virtually everything about an eating disorder resists balanced eating. Explaining elements of body and food science can effectively interrupt and diminish patients' rigid and emotionally charged food/body beliefs and behaviors.

As we'll see later, science know-how also opens a path for patients to grasp and buy into Structured Eating's process. It gives clinicians a path to discuss the body without the eating disorder's distorting filters. Perhaps most important, science makes plain to patients how and why eating within the structure *benefits* their bodies and their ability to function during a day.

Structured Eating provides a degree of safety for patients and fosters the yoga tenet of *ahimsa* (non-violence), while learning practices that (eventually) look honestly and compassionately at the ways that we cause aggression or harm to ourselves or others. Yoga gives clinicians concrete, foundational tools to help patients inhabit and navigate their bodies through Structured Eating's practice of what, when, and how much to eat.

We believe that providers must be advocates for the client's body throughout treatment. That role is especially crucial during Structured Eating, when the patient's capacity for self-advocacy is limited. As this patient recalls:

> I spent my time at home looking in the mirror, counting calories, working out behind closed doors, or sleeping because I was fatigued (due to malnutrition). I must admit that I was in extreme denial about all these thoughts and behaviors until my parents became so alarmed that they got an eating disorder treatment team for me. I kept on losing weight, and dropped to my all-time low, which felt like achieving my ultimate goal. In reality, I was stuck in a place I could not get out of myself; I was in too deep to help myself. Anorexia had taken over my mind and body. I was sent for an evaluation at a hospital-based eating disorder treatment center and started the next day. I remember feeling like I wasn't sick enough to be there and was honestly surprised that they took me as a patient. That shows how extreme denial was in my thought process.

We articulate our advocacy for clients' bodies from the start. When clients rebel against us for "making them eat," we have a clear and extremely practical explanation. Without a strong and sure stance, we risk colluding with the eating disorder:

> You hired me to advocate for your body's needs and because I know about eating disorders. Right now, you're unable to do this on your

own, without an experienced advocate. That's me—working with *you*. I can and will advocate for your body. I can even shop, cook, and eat *with* you, but I can't eat *for* you.

You are hurting your body by not feeding it appropriately. *Together* we need to find ways to treat it better. This meal plan is a way that works; I have science and my experience to back this up. I need you to trust I am here to care for your body in the moments when you cannot.

We expect and accept tension, but our message must stay grounded in truth (what yoga calls *satya*).

My colleague Karen worked with a new client who continued to lose weight after two nutrition sessions. Karen said she was afraid that taking a harder stance might mean this person (already dealing with many other problems, like a loved one's death) never returns to treatment.

Karen and I recognized that the client was unable to gain control of her eating disorder without firm guidance. So, we worked together on how Karen could deliver her boundaries message simply and clearly. She began the next session like this:

> Let's pause for a moment and remember that you came here with a desperate need to get help. It would be a disservice to the health of your body to continue letting the eating disorder hurt your body by dictating how you eat and exercise.
>
> As your body's advocate, let me make clear three things:
>
> 1. Your body needs you to limit exercise.
> 2. You need to see an outpatient psychotherapist to work with your grief.
> 3. Your body and I will give you two weeks to follow our meal plan every day to see if your body can gain weight. If not, we will refer you to a more intensive treatment program.

Of course, the patient argued that she had already added calories and needed her exercise to feel less stressed. Karen persisted, and repeated her body-advocate statements. By the session's end, the patient stopped fighting back, and never threatened to leave treatment. Instead, she seemed relieved to have a line to follow. Later the same day, Karen received an email from the patient saying she had not exercised, and had called a therapist and purchased the recommended supplements.

The Core Components

Because Structured Eating is mechanical and guided, it lays the foundation for upcoming phases. It also lays the groundwork for more integrated life processes. Patients build *from* Structured Eating into Mindful, Intuitive, and

Mastered phases—and, because recovery is seldom linear, we reassure patients that Structured Eating remains their foundation; they don't "regress" to it.

Structured Eating cannot be rushed. A client may take weeks, months, a year, or more to become proficient in the format and practice of structured eating. Time is an asset, not a problem here!

Structured Eating begins to restore hunger and fullness cues through the practice of eating bite after bite until the meal is completed. If a patient in restrictive cycles is full before the meal is completed, we encourage/train them to keep eating until the meal has ended. If a patient in a binge cycle still feels hungry after eating the meal, we encourage/train them to sit with their hunger until the next meal or snack.

The longer a patient practices Structured Eating:

- The better the body learns to communicate effectively with the brain about its nutritional needs.
- The more ingrained becomes the patient's routine of feeding the body what it needs.
- The more practice a body has in sensing and responding to meeting its nutritional needs.
- The more the body can relax in knowing that its needs are being met reliably.

We give the people in our care structured or semi-structured meal plans that include balanced meals and snacks. Restoration of appetite and normal eating begins mechanically, helping the stomach and brain communicate more effectively. It may take several weeks or months before hunger and satiety cues regulate themselves. The *practice* of mechanical eating leads toward regular, balanced eating.

There are three basic components of structured eating:

1. *when* to eat
2. *what* to eat
3. *how much* to eat

How exactly does this work?

When to Eat

Based on the science of circadian rhythms and energy needs, we set two simple and important parameters (or as I call them, sacred suggestions) about when to eat:

1. Eat within the first 30 to 60 minutes of waking up. This ensures that your body moves out of the fasting slumber state and gets vital metabolic energy to start the day. More on the science behind this later!

2. Eat every three to four hours after the initial meal. The complex system of feeding our body, brain waves, blood sugar regulation, etc. demands it!

As patients practice these "sacred suggestions," a pattern of eating develops that allows for structured and sensible placement of what clients learn to call "essential eating events."

- breakfast meal
- morning floating snack
- lunch meal
- mini-meal
- pre-dinner floating snack
- dinner
- evening floating snack.

Most of the time, scheduling the "floating" snack depends on the person's life situation. They may need to eat a balanced snack:

- before breakfast
- between breakfast and lunch
- a few hours after lunch
- a few hours before dinner
- a few hours after dinner.

Every eating event is a balanced compilation of food. The three "traditional" meals have the largest amount of food. The one mini-meal has a little bit less. The multiple *floating* snacks have less than the mini-meal. Making this framework explicit sets important expectations for the patient and the dietitian:

- The meals and mini-meal are not optional.
- The snacks are not optional, but they can "float" to meet the patient's schedule and other needs.
- Each eating event includes timely packages of foods.
- Your body urgently needs you to follow the process.

What to Eat

Each timely package of food contains some amount of four essential macronutrients:

- complex carbohydrates
- proteins
- fats
- fruits and/or vegetables.

Much of what patients "know" about these foods are usually myths, misinformation, and mistaken/distorted eating disorder beliefs or stories. We respond to the distortion with science and, when necessary, good old common sense. We educate, listen, and respond. And then, we repeat.

We do this through simple, concrete questions, like: What do you usually eat for breakfast? Depending on the diagnosis and/or symptoms, we hear answers like this:

- I had a half-cup of fat-free, sugar-free, lactose-free yogurt with two pineapple chunks. I sprinkled a teaspoon of Fiber One cereal on top (anorexia, bulimia, binge eating disorder with chronic weight-loss dieting, other specified feeding or eating disorder (OSFED)).
- I didn't have breakfast (anorexia, bulimia, binge eating disorder with chronic weight-loss dieting, OSFED, avoidant restrictive food intake disorder (ARFID)).
- I had a Cinnabon and coffee (binge eating disorder, bulimia, OSFED).

Next, we ask: what do you know about these foods? Can you tell me where a cinnamon bun falls in the categories of essential macronutrients and describe what that macronutrient does in your body? We hear answers like this:

It's a carb. And a carbohydrate is something with no nutrients. It's all sugar and it turns into fat.

We (matter-of-factly) respond with the scientific fact that the body turns carbohydrates into glucose, not fat—and that glucose/sugar is the *only* source of energy for the brain.

Concrete data like this help clinician and patient to bring meal plans to life. (As you'll see, our meal plans don't feature non-fat yogurt, abstinence, or Cinnabon-only meals.)

By the way, we are nutrition-neutral about how people get their carbohydrates, proteins, fats, fruits, and vegetables. Because of geography and/or income level, people in many parts of the United States and beyond can't access the same variety of food (e.g., fresh produce and organic whole grains) as other people. Too often, patients, dietitians, and others identify—explicitly or subconsciously—foods like fresh produce and organic whole grain as "healthier" and/or "better" foods. Let's vigorously examine and challenge our food stereotypes and biases as clinicians. If we don't:

1. Eating disorders will manipulate our food stereotypes and biases.
2. We're disserving our patients.

Please avoid expressing (or holding) judgmental beliefs and attitudes about frozen vegetables, "white" bread, ballpark hot dogs, canned fruit, chocolate milk, farmer's market produce, grass-fed beef, or raw-milk yogurt. Here's why:

1. Regardless of the purchase price, every one of those eight foods breaks down into essential macronutrients.
2. Regardless of their zip code or wallet, every person with an eating disorder deserves treatment, understanding, and respect.

Complex carbohydrates come from foods like grains or starches. A serving of complex carbohydrates equals approximately:

- one slice of bread
- one half-cup of cooked grain or pasta
- a small potato
- three-quarters to one cup of cereal.

Depending on our clinical goals, we usually aim to consume one to three servings of carbohydrates per meal.

Proteins come from animal and non-animal sources. A serving is approximately:

- three ounces of animal protein (e.g., fish, poultry, beef, pork)
- three-quarters cup of beans and legumes
- one large or two small eggs
- one ounce of cheese, one cup of yogurt or milk, or one half-cup cottage cheese.

Depending on our clinical goals, we usually aim to consume one to two servings of protein per meal.

Fats come from foods like oil, butter, avocado, mayonnaise, and salad dressings. Fats are primarily made up of lipids or fatty acids. A serving is:

- about two teaspoons of oil
- one tablespoon of mayonnaise or salad dressing
- one-eighth of an avocado
- two teaspoons of butter.

In a moderate meal, we typically will consume two to three servings of a fat.

Fruits and vegetables come from (surprise!) fruits and vegetables. They have fiber, water, and high concentrations of vitamins and minerals. We generally measure a serving as:

- one piece of fresh fruit
- one cup cut fruit or vegetable
- one half-cup cooked fruit or vegetable
- one quarter-cup dried fruit.

The inclusion of these food groups creates what nutritionists call "balanced eating." Balanced eating doesn't necessarily mean consuming *equal amounts* of each macronutrient during the eating event. Instead, the goal is consuming *adequate amounts* of each macronutrient, so the body gets the nourishment it needs *when* it needs that nourishment.

In Structured Eating:

- *Meals* are balanced with the four essential macronutrients: complex carbohydrates, proteins, fats, fruits and/or vegetables.
- *Mini-meals* are about half to three-quarters the size of a meal—and still contain the four essential macronutrients: complex carbohydrates, proteins, fats, fruits and/or vegetables.
- *Snacks* are smaller food packets than mini-meals. They pair a food with *both* protein and fat (e.g., a hard-boiled egg or cheese) with fruit, vegetable, or complex carbohydrate:

  1.   protein and fat + fruit
  2.   protein and fat + vegetable
  3.   protein and fat + complex carbohydrate.

We'll get into more detail about portion sizes later, but to give you a rough idea of what a person with bulimia eats during three balanced, well-portioned "traditional" meals in Structured Eating:

- breakfast: one cup of oatmeal, with one quarter-cup of nuts, one quarter-cup of raisins, and one cup of milk
- lunch: a turkey and cheese sandwich with avocado, lettuce, and tomato and an apple
- dinner: shrimp stir fry with four ounces of shrimp, a cup of rice, and one and a half cups of cooked vegetables with two teaspoons of sesame oil.

"Snack" is often a hard concept for clients to grasp. We often address this problem by asking: "What isn't a snack?" Mass marketing and our cultural eating norms seldom differentiate between "*snacking*" and "*dessert*." Clients need to understand what these terms mean in Structured Eating and for their body.

- *Snacking*: There is nothing inherently wrong with "*snacking*," but we need to recognize noshing, grazing, and so on, as *behaviors*, rather than "eating events." There is certainly room in a recovered diet for a few pretzels (as opposed to one pretzel or 150 pretzels) before dinner. Fortunately,

Structured Eating trains patients to understand that eating disorder "snack-ing" *behavior* rarely results in a balanced eating event. Disordered snacking *behavior* lacks mindfulness and, therefore, is a problematic symptom.

- *Dessert:* Dessert is not inherently bad or unhealthy. However, Struc-tured Eating trains patients to distinguish between dessert and snack. (They are not interchangeable.) Foods like ice cream, cake, or cookies accompany a balanced meal. A cookie by itself at 4:00 pm isn't a balanced, recovery-oriented eating event.

When it comes to meeting the body's needs, an eating event is incomplete if it includes only a piece of fruit, a granola bar, or a bag of popcorn.

Let's illustrate with three common food items: bread, peanut butter, and banana.

- meal: sandwich with two pieces of bread and two tablespoons of peanut butter, with the banana on the side (or sliced up inside the sandwich, if you're like Elvis Presley)
- mini-meal: one slice of bread with one tablespoon of peanut butter, and half of a banana
- snack: one small banana and one tablespoon of peanut butter

Each of these eating events is balanced and, therefore, gives the body the energy and nutrition it wants and needs.

Of course, someone must shop, prepare, and/or cook for each eating event. Many of our patients do not shop, prepare, and/or cook food. They (literally) may not know how to perform those skills, or else their eating disorder "prohibits" using those skills.

We must teach people in our care:

- How and what to shop for. We take our clients to grocery stores to show them what to buy and support them *while* they buy. We show clients how to make and submit online grocery orders, with choices that fit the meal plan.
- How to prepare food. Whether we teach clients how to make dinner or not, prepare to answer questions factually and without condescen-sion. For example:
  - Which pot do I use for pasta?
  - How do I boil water?
  - How much oil do I add?
  - How do you peel a potato?
  - How much water do I need to boil potatoes (or pasta or eggs, etc.)?
  - What's the best method for cooking a chicken (or hamburger, or eggs, etc.)?
  - Do I eat *this* part of the chicken (or broccoli, or eggs, etc.)?

We spend many sessions giving recipes and taking our clients through the process of cooking.

How Much to Eat

We assess how much our patients need to eat based on many factors, including: their weight, symptoms, nutritional status, and metabolic state. Dietitians use these factors to create a meal plan to address the patient's needs and treatment goals.

We must strike a balance between staying directive enough that patients learn how to prepare their meals and open-minded enough to decrease patient overthinking. Navigating the balance requires vigilance about how eating disorders distort and control thinking—and cunningly redefine and mis-define simple words like "servings."

Of course, we can't completely abandon words like "serving" which are central to our profession. Integrated Eating dietitians say "serving" less often than dietitians outside eating disorders treatment. Our go-to word (and concept) is *ratio* (ratio of food components in an eating event), which helps defuse conversations (read: arguments) about terms. Ratio also supports the directive–open balance we're seeking.

Traditionally, dietitians who specialize in disordered eating have a host of eating/nutrition goals and approaches when preparing meal plans. In the Integrated Eating approach, we designate one of three meal plan goals:

1. weight restoration
2. weight maintenance
3. metabolic balance.

As treatment continues, we may stay with one clinical goal and/or shift to another one (more on this below).

We frame each meal and snack in terms of the *ratio* of food amount (or portion) for each of the four micronutrient categories. For example, a meal ratio of 3:2:1:2 represents:

- *three* servings of complex carbohydrates
- *two* servings of protein
- *one* serving of fat
- *two* servings of fruit and/or vegetables.

Regardless of clinical goals, our meal plans have some variation and flexibility. They all serve to navigate both provider and patient through the food recovery journey. (The next two chapters will show specific meal plans and serving ratios in action.)

Reader Thought Experiment

Imagine you woke up hungry at 7:30 this morning and decide to eat a bagel with butter at 8:00. Your body wants to eat within an hour of awakening. You did that (score!), but your meal lacks protein, fruit, or vegetables. This "unbalanced" meal doesn't supply the fuel (nutrition) your body needs. You are starving at 9:30 and (instead of waiting for lunch), you raid the work pantry and eat one or two pastries left over from yesterday's meeting.

For lunch, you decide on a salad with chicken to catch up on protein (because you haven't eaten any yet). You forget to add any complex carbohydrates (like bread). By mid-afternoon, you're craving the carbs your lunch lacked, so you grab a giant chocolate chip cookie.

By dinnertime, you're not hungry, so you eat a light dinner, or skip it altogether. Then, an hour or so later, you get super-hungry. So, you drive to a Korean takeout for beef and broccoli with white rice, go back home, and eat until you're over-full.

Now, convinced that you've irrevocably blown your "nutritional day," you dig into a pint of ice-cream to ease your guilt.

Write down your responses to these thought experiment questions and reflections:

1. Conceptualize and/or perceive your eating:

    a) Did you see your food consumption as "eating events"?
    b) How (if at all) did you differentiate between "snack" and "meals"?
    c) Which eating event (if any) seemed like a mini-meal?
    d) On reflection, which time of day would have worked best for a mini-meal?

2. Consider any disruption of: *when* to eat, *what* to eat, *how much* to eat:

    a) at breakfast (what to eat)
    b) morning snack (when to eat, what to eat)
    c) lunch (what to eat)
    d) afternoon snack (what to eat)
    e) dinner (when to eat, how much to eat)
    f) evening snack (when to eat, what to eat).

Now imagine experiencing this eating day in the dysregulated, malnourished body and mind of someone with an eating disorder.

Next, let's rewrite the story as if you are practicing Structured Eating.

Imagine you woke up hungry at 7:30 and remember that your body needs to eat within the first hour. You decide to eat a bagel with butter at 8:00. But first, you review your meal plan. It shows that you missed two balanced meal elements: protein and fruit or vegetables. Instead of butter, you put peanut butter (which has protein *and* fat) on the bagel and eat some apple slices. This meal keeps you satiated until lunchtime.

At noon, you order your favorite salad chock full of chicken, avocado, chickpeas, and vinaigrette. To create balance, you also say "yes" to the side roll. You finish lunch with a small piece of dark chocolate. After lunch you're fired up and engaged all afternoon.

By 3:30 or 4:00 pm, you feel your energy dip, check the clock, and seize the moment for a quick stretch and afternoon snack. You check the pantry and grab yogurt, raisins, and granola to make a balanced parfait.

After work, you run a few errands on your way home. At the grocery store, you choose hamburger, buns, and frozen spinach for dinner. Once home, you fry a burger, toast the bun, boil the spinach, and eat a satisfying meal.

A few hours later, you're in the mood for a treat and have a few Graham crackers with a tall glass of cold milk. At the end of the day, you reflect on how helpful it was to stay on a schedule for eating, how satisfying balanced eating is, and how easy it was to eat moderately. You resolve to do it again tomorrow!

Structured Eating brings concrete, useful, and desirable results. So, why do people with eating disorders have such a hard time doing it?

Resistance

As with other elements of eating disorders treatment, resistance to Structured Eating is common. Exploring resistance with the patient helps get them on board. We want to learn where the patient is starting from: their eating history, their current eating patterns, and their symptoms.

A matter-of-fact, non-didactic conversational tone helps to reduce resistance tension—and share some reality about the science of nourishing the body. Here's an example:

> Just so you know, we nutritionists/dietitians didn't invent this whole thing about meals, circadian rhythms, brain waves, metabolism, blood sugar, and how the body works. I'm just a scientist just telling you what's real.
>
> The human body is not a manufactured device, like a sewing machine or space station. From day one, the body's "wiring" operates to meet our needs before and after we get up with the sun and go to sleep with the stars.
>
> Think of how an infant's body is wired to sleep more at night than during the day … and to eat every few hours until full. The baby "automatically" functions in structured eating mode. And it works! The baby survives, grows, and keeps eating until full.

I've studied the science for years, so you can trust me on this. Science proves what the body already knows:

- *when* we need energy
- the *rate* that we need energy during the day
- *what* categories of nourishment provide that energy.

A resistant patient will say things like:

> I just can't eat more than half of an orange in the morning. I'm not allowed to. And if I did, I'd be completely bloated, be in a panic, and obsess about it all day long. I can't live like that!

We reply with short, simple questions, such as: "Can you add yogurt to your half-orange this week?" We immediately begin using science to support our question.

- A piece of fruit alone doesn't give your body what it needs when you wake up. Your body needs each macronutrient: complex carbohydrates, proteins, fats, fruits and vegetables; what we call a balanced meal.
- Your body is in a fasting state during sleep. Its metabolism slows down to conserve energy like a hibernating bear.
- Once we wake up, our body's metabolism instinctively revs up and uses more energy.

Science measures the body's energy consumption in units called calories. However, eating disorders (and much of our culture) consistently distort and pervert the "calorie" word. One resistance-reduction strategy is to explain the science with alternative metaphors and terminology.

We might ask a patient with restrictive behaviors to imagine their body as a North Dakota office building. Its furnace has the potential to heat every room to 80 degrees. To do that, the furnace needs four cubic feet of natural gas every hour.

On winter nights, the thermostat sets back to 45 degrees, so the water pipes don't freeze and burst. From 9:00 at night until 7:00 the next morning, the furnace needs only half a cubic foot of natural gas per hour.

During the day, the people and equipment (computers, copiers, phone and data networks, etc.) work most comfortably and efficiently with the thermostat set at 70. The furnace consumes three cubic feet of gas per hour to maintain this "optimal" warmth: 70 degrees.

But what happens if only one cubic foot of gas gets through the supply pipe during the day? The inside temperature drops to 55. The building and its occupants enter a cold and inefficient state. The equipment acts up.

The people are distracted and accomplish less. The furnace sputters and can't keep up with the needs signaled by the thermostat.

In your "office building" body, food is the natural gas, your metabolism is the furnace, the thermostat is your brain, and the people, computers, copiers, phone and data networks, etc. are your internal organs and systems. If you don't supply enough fuel, your body:

- cannot reach or use its optimal energy
- operates in a sub-optimal state that saps your ability to do what you need and want to do
- operates in a sub-optimal state that, if continued over time, damages your brain, organs, and metabolism.

Patients need to hear that:

- If I eat a balanced meal, I assist my body to generate energy to do things I *need* to do and *want* to do.
- If I don't eat a balanced meal, I'm making a decision to keep my body in a sub-optimal state. I will not have energy to do things I *need* to do and *want* to do.

Given the nature of eating disorders, some patients won't care: "So what? I'll stay in a fasting state. I'll just wait until I'm really hungry or until I really can't stand not eating." Meeting the patient where they are, we lean into parts of them (or their eating disorder) that value metabolism's role. In other words, we use the metabolism to our (and their) advantage.

I usually explore this with a question like: "Tell me what you believe metabolism is." Patients might honestly say: "It's what keeps me fat," or "It's what helps me lose weight." Or, they might say what they think I want to hear. Either response lets us dig into the science of what metabolism is and what it isn't.

> Metabolism is how the body uses energy to do what it needs to do, like breathe, think, and walk. Science proves that the body's metabolism is disrupted by restricting, bingeing, purging, and other erratic eating patterns. It is *also* disrupted by trauma, depression, anxiety, and addiction. Necessary medications can disrupt metabolism, too (although, that's *not* a reason to stop taking them). The disruption decreases the chances your body is utilizing energy optimally.

> On the other hand, science proves that when your body's metabolism runs optimally, the rest of your body runs better, and serves you better, too. You are likely to feel more energy, think more clearly, and have more stable moods.

Science has also proven what it takes to restore disrupted metabolism: structured eating, movement, or rest (depending on how much energy you're using), balanced sleep, hygiene and healthy stress management.

Let's say the patient continues to resist. We acknowledge that their thoughts and fears are real. We explain that their resistance is not unusual; after many years of working with eating disorders, their thoughts and fears don't surprise us.

But we also articulate our belief about what brought them here to our office. In order to plow through the resistance, we must coach and cheer lead for the patient's recovery. I will say:

> Well, you are here with me—which means that there is a part of you that wants to recover.
>
> I'm a nutritionist who works with people with eating disorders. Your eating disorder is real. I understand that it believes (and tells you) that you can't do more. I also understand that *other* parts of you feel differently. Right now, those parts may take up less space than the eating disorder. They may be shrouded, covered, or weak. But those other parts are also real, and they really exist. And I believe you wouldn't be here with me if *no part of you* can do more.
>
> So, tell me where that part of you is in your body, mind, soul, or spirit. And tell me what *that part of you* is willing to do today and what commitment it's willing to make for your recovery.

We know that an eating disorder can be so entrenched that the patient can't conceive of doing Structured Eating. We forthrightly respond with more science:

> Look, I hear what you're saying. I know that there is a part of you that wants to give your body the food it needs, but part of you is *not capable of* doing it. My education and experience tell me that we need to get you into a higher level of care, where you have more meal support.

When patients are afraid of hospitalization or inpatient treatment, we explicitly acknowledge it.

> We know this is very hard for you. We also know that some part of you understands that this work is hard—maybe the hardest thing you'll ever do in your life. Remember, your eating disorder is real. We're asking for your commitment to do this. To stay out of a higher level of care, you must start to feed your body in a way that it deserves. If you can't do it, that tells us you need more support than you're getting now.

By coming here, you've appointed me, your nutritionist, to advocate for your body because—right now—you can't find a voice to advocate for your body on your own. It may *feel* like you and I are battling over a half-cup of yogurt, but in reality, I'm voicing your body's needs. Your body needs to eat balanced meals. This is what recovery is asking of you right now, today.

We know how scary that can be—and we will support you. We will hold hope for you when you can't. With experience, my patients (and I) eventually recognize that our fears are usually bigger than the reality. I also see an important reality about *you*: part of you wants to recover; otherwise you wouldn't be here. One bite at a time is OK in Structured Eating; it works.

At the same time, my support and expectations are firm. One bite at a time doesn't mean we're going soft or letting you off the hook. We expect completion of each meal and snack.

What People Don't Tell You About Eating This Way

Think about an old car sitting for years in the driveway. When you first try to start it up, the engine may not turn over. You might have to fix some things first. Once you get it to start, the tailpipe may spew out blue smoke and foul odors. The engine will run rough and stall often. But, after more repairs and use, the car starts operating more smoothly and efficiently.

When patients practice Structured Eating after years of disordered eating, their bodies often take a while to get all cylinders running. They may "stall" occasionally, producing unexpected (and sometimes embarrassing) "by-products" like flatulence, bloating, and belching. We expect this and respond (matter-of-factly) by using Integrated Eating's science and yoga threads. Here are some examples:

Flatulence

When you eat chaotically, your body makes fewer digestive enzymes. Your digestive system operates on supply and demand, so your digestive enzyme output takes a while to catch up with your new eating patterns. When you start eating balanced meals, the enzyme shortage means your body won't digest food completely (which leads to what dietitians and physicians call delayed gastric emptying). The not-fully-digested food stays in the gut longer, ferments, and creates gas which must find its way out. You're farting because of enzyme shortage. The enzymes will eventually catch up, so flatulence, too, shall pass (pun intended). To ease your discomfort in the meantime, we can use yoga, a digestive enzyme supplement, and/or probiotics. In fact, yoga has a wind-releasing pose to release trapped gas.

Bloating

Excess air in the belly (known as distension) is also caused by delayed gastric emptying, deficient enzymes, and food fermentation in the gut. Malnutrition can cause dehydration. Balanced eating is the remedy for dehydration, and can cause temporary water retention (as your body's cells adjust). Get your comfy pajamas out and/or do yoga to ease the discomfort.

Belching

Delayed gastric emptying can also cause belching and acid reflux in early recovery. If you stay on your meal plan, structured and timely eating will help the body digest foods more efficiently, which usually means less acid migrating up into the esophagus.

The Upside People Don't Tell You About Eating This Way

Along with telling patients about uncomfortable or embarrassing possibilities, we prepare them for the positive outcomes they are likely to experience during Structured Eating—like increased and/or longer-lasting energy, greater ability to concentrate, and other concrete rewards.

For instance, we use science to explain that, whether the client feels over-full or not full enough, their body is going to be thrilled with the fuel.

> Yes, Structured Eating provides a little bit more food or little bit less food than you usually give your body. And, I guarantee that your body will know how to use the fuel to produce energy. You can trust that your body will use the energy the way it needs to.

I think of a patient with trauma history. Part of her safety net is being radically consumed with weight—so she isn't following her meal plan. My response recognizes and is sensitive to her intense need to be safe and feel safe.

When she ate a "nutrition" bar or smoothie every day for lunch, I pushed her hard to substitute a real food. She feels safer when I suggest simple and doable strategies like: "I give you the authority to get a lunch that is a small sandwich with the same number of calories as the bar. Let's start there." I want her to feel (and, ultimately. to trust) the difference in her body, and build from there.

I explained how real food (like a sandwich) has a longer "transit time" and more whole macronutrients than a "nutrition" bar or smoothie does (e.g., "nutrition" bars have pre-digested macronutrients). A 400-calorie sandwich is a food "brick" for the stomach to mechanically digest. This slower "transit time" allows the body to absorb nutrients more steadily and efficiently. Blood sugar levels will be more stable, she will feel more satisfied, and her energy will be steadier, more consistent, and last longer. By contrast, a 400-calorie smoothie's viscous liquid has a much shorter "transit time" in the stomach.

These elementary examples help us show patients that our bodies are literally made to do this meal thing. Fortunately, science gives us more human biology data to prove that eating a meal every few hours helps our bodies operate better than eating only one, two, or three times a day.

For instance, when food enters the stomach, the stomach stretches. That activates the digestive system's proprioceptors and stretch receptors to signal the medulla oblongata (aka, vagus nerve). The vagus nerve signals back, triggering the stomach's gastric glands to secrete gastric juices we need for digestion. Synergy within the digestive system determines how our bodies assimilate the food.

My patient finally substituted real food for her bar—but only three days a week. Still, she reported: "You know, I can't dispute that on the days I ate the sandwich, I was able to go for a few more hours and could concentrate better." Her body knows the difference. And she can begin to *trust* that her body knows the difference.

Yes, "trusting my body" is a radical idea for someone with an eating disorder. Nevertheless, it is rational, and it works—when we impose the structure! To be clear, adding the sandwich is not an end point. It is an opening that paves the way for us to work on appropriate amounts of balanced food during all eating events—and to practice embodiment.

Structured Eating gives people opportunities—sensations, really—to begin making the connection between balanced nutrition and embodied outcomes like energy and concentration.

I use myself as an example. Because I see three patients in a row, I can't stop every five minutes to eat. Some days, I have evening sessions, so I can't have a traditionally timed dinner. In each scenario, when I *do* eat, I need to know that the food will fuel enough energy to last long enough to do my job well.

Inviting my patient to reflect on her afternoon experience is helping her connect these ideas to *her* life. I said: "Maybe you don't feel hunger signals in mid-afternoon, but you can't deny that you feel exhausted around 3 pm." That's an opening to explain that everyone's body has physiologic shifts every day between 2:00 and 4:00 pm. Our bodies transition from a peak energy plateau at midday toward a gradual, natural energy slow-down, using fewer calories per hour as the body prepares to sleep, like a thermostat dialing back the furnace at night.

Combining the science of circadian rhythms and energy use with their own experience of daily energy fluctuation makes a powerful case for Structured Eating. When we use neutral language and labels for "problem" times of day, patients are more likely to buy into the notion that eating isn't optional. We need balanced and appropriately scheduled eating to concentrate, focus, and help our bodies move successfully from nourishing breakfast to nourishing sleep.

Navigating the Process

Structured Eating accommodates flexibility but requires a *firm* approach. For example, a client can float their snack, choose their breakfast protein, *and* we still expect them to finish it.

After all, few of us wake up with the sun and sleep with the stars, like our ancestors did. I have a patient who gets up at 4:30 am to practice yoga before she goes to work. She cannot eat a full meal that early, so she has a balanced floating snack before yoga and breakfast afterward. Another patient has breakfast at 7:00, but no free period at school until 2:00 pm. So, she needs a mid-morning snack to maintain her energy and focus.

Some patients ask us to show them how to eat: "All right, I guess I could eat half a cup of yogurt for breakfast with my orange. But that's going to be very scary. Could you show me or do it with me?"

We address those concerns by role-playing the situation. Or, we invite them to text a picture of the orange and yogurt before they eat, so we can see how it looks on the plate. We then determine whether it's too much or too little—and respond with our feedback. As I write this in New York, one of my patients is texting me photos of all her day's meals from Kenya.

In addition, our staff provide in-person meal support beyond the regular nutrition session. A patient can schedule eating events with a dietitian or meal coach in our offices, at a restaurant, or at their home—getting real-time support on how to portion, eat, etc.

Many people with bulimia and/or binge eating disorder have more regular contact and interaction with food than someone with restrictive anorexia. For these patients, Structured Eating (and meal support) is usually about balance, balance, balance.

Some patients with eating disorders show orthorexic tendencies, eating nothing but "natural" foods. I think of a patient who explained that she ate yogurt with nuts every morning. I inquired about the portions and acknowledged that her current breakfast seemed relatively balanced. When I asked if she could add some fresh fruit, she agreed.

Then, I asked what else she ate for breakfast. She said yogurt with nuts *every* morning. As a clinician, the Structured Eating conversation doesn't end at "OK, you have a balanced breakfast."

I pushed on and asked her to consider having something like an English muffin with cheese instead of yogurt and nuts some mornings. She instantly and adamantly insisted that she doesn't eat cheese or store-bought bread products because they're processed.

I then introduced the "rotating three" concept to build balance and variety into Structured Eating over multiple days (more on this in later chapters). Ideally, the rotation variety plants seeds for learning food flexibility. Together, we created a structure of:

- three breakfasts (which include cheese and bread)
- three lunches
- three dinners
- six snacks/mini-meals.

On Monday she chooses one of the three options for each meal and two of the six options for snacks/mini-meals. This works even when a patient feels afraid and/or rigid. They can take a one, two, three … one, two, three … one, two, three approach, and still accomplish balance and variety. They can rotate more loosely, and that works, too.

Many binge eaters restrict during the day and binge at night. So, we discuss the science of what happens to energy and concentration when they don't eat balanced foods every few hours.

> Eating balanced foods at breakfast, mid-morning, lunch, mid-afternoon, etc. ensures that your body is more fed—which means you have more protection around binge eating *later* in the day. You may binge, but binge less frequently, and/or find yourself eating different types and amounts of food. But I predict you will see changes at night if you take care of your nutritional needs during the day.

These conversations often gain traction because many binge eaters urgently want their symptoms to decrease. Many people with bulimia and/or binge eating disorder say that, by the time they're seeing me, they're very scared and feel very out of control.

Of course, many of these patients fear that they will be—or feel— deprived during Structured Eating. "What you put on my meal plan isn't going to be enough!" I usually respond by saying:

> You may *feel* like you are deprived. We can explore the parts of you that feel deprived when your body gets sufficient food. However, just so you know, if you eat this amount, your body will get the energy it needs today.

Balanced eating often includes spacing between eating events. I have a middle-aged patient who compulsively eats four to six times between lunch and dinner. So, we're working on spacing out the time between their eating events. Yes, for now, they can have three snacks between lunch and dinner, but we space at least an hour and a half between snacks. They're using a simple timing technique. Right after lunch, they set their smartphone alarm for 90 minutes. Then, right after the first snack, they set it for another 90 minutes. Because they want so badly for their symptoms to end, they are willing to tolerate the discomfort while waiting for the alarm. They report that the experiment is helping them reframe how they think about what it means to eat during the day.

We *Are* Asking a Lot

Structured Eating asks our patients to put mind over matter, and to eat regardless of state, feeling, or mood.

When patients arrive, their lives are like a chaotic ball of different-colored yarns. We ask them to pull out and separate the emotional and nutritional yarns. Structured Eating is like a knitting pattern. We know that the eating disorder's "static electricity" draws the emotional and nutritional threads toward one other, but we don't want them to get or stay tangled up. When they do tangle, we stabilize the nutrition thread before dealing with emotional eating behaviors.

When we can tolerate our feelings without acting on them with food or how we eat, it's like holding one thread taut while knitting and purling a second thread. Just as we must follow a pattern to finish knitting a wool scarf, we must follow Structured Eating to create our recovery. When we witness our feelings mindfully, label them, are with them, we begin to dissipate the eating disorder's "static electricity" by grounding our eating.

Now, if any part of our Structured Eating discussion sounds simplistic, naive, or too good to be true, remember this:

Integrated Eating providers are realistic. We expect Structured Eating to be hard and uncomfortable. We expect eating disorder "voices" and sensations to erupt and attack the recovery process. Whether people seek treatment or not, they get a lot of crap from their eating disorder all day, every day.

I tell my patients:

> Structured Eating is not about how you *feel*. This is about what *you do* and what *you don't do* to meet the needs of your malnourished, unbalanced body. Right now, you need to do Structured Eating. Your eating disorder creates intense reactions because it can't survive without holding you in its grip. Its original intention was to protect you, but now it doesn't want to let go of you.

> Recovered people tell me that Structured Eating was where and how they learned to say: "No more!" and began to battle the eating disorder. Eventually their authentic self emerged victorious. Once we're through this structured phase of feeding your body, you can (and will) have conversations about how you feel. In the meantime, our work is about what you do.

In Structured Eating, our patients are beginners, using elementary, foundational tools to find ways through the eating disorder's resistance. We expect them to use those tools and build on their foundation. Next, we'll explore the details of putting Structured Eating to work in real life.

Bibliography

Buchhorn, R., Hauk, F., Kertess-Szlaninka, T., Dippacher, S., and Willaschek, C. (2016). The impact of nutrition on the autonomic nervous system. A model for eating disorders in childhood. *International Journal of Food and Nutritional Science*, 3(1), 585–606.

Carreiro, A.L., Dhillon, J., Gordon, S., Higgins, K.A., Jacobs, A.G., McArthur, B. M., and Mattes, R.D. (2016). The Macronutrients, appetite, and energy intake. *Annual Review of Nutrition*, 36, 73–103.

Costin, C. and Kelly, J. (Eds.). *Yoga and Eating Disorders* (New York: Routledge, 2016).

El Ghoch, M., Calugi, S., Lamburghini, S., and Dalle Grave, R. (2014). Anorexia nervosa and body fat distribution: A systematic review. *Nutrients*, 6(9), 3895–3912.

Kinzig, K.P., Coughlin, J.W., et al. (2007). Insulin, glucose, and pancreatic poly-peptide responses to a test meal in restricting type anorexia nervosa before and after weight restoration. *American Journal of Physiology-Endocrinology and Metabolism*, 292(5), E1441–E1446.

La Bounty, P.M., Campbell, B.I., et al. (2011). International Society of Sports Nutrition position stand: Meal frequency. *Journal of the International Society of Sports Nutrition*, 8, 4.

Marzola, E., Nasser, J.A., Hashim, S.A., Shih, P.A., and Kaye, W.H. (2013). Nutritional rehabilitation in anorexia nervosa: Review of the literature and implications for treatment. *BMC Psychiatry*, 13, 290.

Mayer, E.A. (2011). Gut feelings: The emerging biology of gut-brain communication. *National Review of Neuroscience*, 12(8), 453–466.

Mergenthaler, P., Lindauer, U., Dienel, G.A., and Meisel, A. (2013). Sugar for the brain: The role of glucose in physiological and pathological brain function. *Trends in Neurosciences*, 36(10), 587–597.

Purves, D., Augustine, G.J., et al. (Ed.). Mechanoreceptors specialized for proprio-ception. In *Neuroscience*. 6th Edition. (Sunderland, MA: Sinauer Associates, 2017), 169-198.

Sato, Y. and Fukudo, S. (2015). Gastrointestinal symptoms and disorders in patients with eating disorders. *Clinical Journal of Gastroenterology*, 8(4), 255–263.

Scribner Reiter, C. and Graves, L. (2010). Nutrition therapy for eating disorders. *Eating and Feeding Disorders*, 25(2), 122–136.

Skerrett, P.J. and Willett, W.C. (2010). Essentials of healthy eating: A guide. *Journal of Midwifery & Women's Health*, 55(6), 492–501.

Smeets, P.A., Erkner, A., and de Graaf, C. (2010). Cephalic phase responses and appetite. *Nutrition Reviews*, 68(11), 643–655.

Touger-Decker, R. and Mobley, S. (2013). Position of the American Dietetic Association: Nutrition intervention in the treatment of eating disorders. *Journal of the American of Nutrition and Dietetics*, 113(5), 639–701.

Zitting, K.-M., Vujovic, N., et al. (2018). Human resting energy expenditure varies with circadian phase. *Current Biology*, 28(22), 3523–3710. R1283–R1324.

3 Structured Eating in Real Life
Morning

Before diving into the details of organizing a day's five or six eating events, let's tackle a skill which patients need for *every* eating event: planning. In some ways, it's like the order of operations in math: calculate the numbers in the wrong order, and your answer doesn't reflect reality!

After living with their illness (often for many years), many of our patients know only the eating disorder's "order of operations." To nourish their body, patients must practice and learn the order of each new-to-them eating operation.

During structured eating, our patients need a lot of support and hands-on modeling, just like when they learned multiplication and division. They may attend a meal support group and/or eat out at a restaurant with the meal support group. A dietitian or eating disorder-trained coach can help the patient learn shopping and cooking skills. We often demonstrate and/or explain how to make rice, pasta, or sautéed vegetables.

"Please Excuse My Dear Aunt Sally"

While those cooking operations may be obvious to us (doh!), a patient's "I don't know how to boil water" dilemma shows how profoundly eating disorders distort and diminish people's lives. They also harm people's ability to take care of their basic needs.

Recovery from an eating disorder is exponentially more difficult than learning the algebraic mnemonic "Please Excuse My Dear Aunt Sally" for parentheses, exponents, multiplication/division, addition/subtraction.

Any time we can break the "how to, how many, and what kind" process into step-by-step chunks (like math teachers do), we help our patients reacquaint themselves with food, eating, and body restoration.

Here's Structured Eating order of operations:

- Dietitian and patient discuss their clinical and nutritional goals.
- Dietitian and patient lay out the meal plan together.
- Dietitian and patient lay out menus, food combinations, and options.

- Dietitian and patient examine the patient's schedule and fit eating events within the schedule.
- Patient decides on one or more methods to meet the meal plan:

  1. Prepare at home: these foods are fresh, frozen, or a mixture of the two. For instance, fresh fish, vegetables, and raw potatoes or frozen chicken stir fry with frozen brown rice.
  2. Assembled somewhere else: store-bought foods to eat or combine with other foods at home. For example, getting a rotisserie chicken and pairing it with frozen mixed veggies and microwaved mac and cheese.
  3. Order/pick-up: foods made to order at a restaurant. This can include many cuisines, from sushi and burgers to lasagne and pad thai.

- Patient learns how and where to purchase *meal plan* foodstuffs at a grocery:

  1. how to create a grocery shopping list
  2. locating stores that carry foods needed for the meal plan
  3. obtaining transportation to and from the grocery or groceries.

- Patient learns where and when to purchase ready-to-eat and/or made-to-order *meal plan* food at a restaurant, café, bodega, convenience store, etc.:

  1. researching and locating businesses that sell ready-to-eat and/or made-to-order *meal plan* food
  2. obtaining transportation to and/or from businesses that sell ready-to-eat and/or made-to-order *meal plan* food.

- Patient learns how to prepare store-bought ingredients, so they become a meal, mini-meal, and/or snack.

  1. practicing basic skills, such as storing foods so they remain fresh, boiling, sautéing, broiling, baking, microwaving, grilling, blending, roasting, etc.
  2. choosing, practicing, and completing recipes
  3. choosing recipes to reuse, based on data from step two
  4. continue choosing, practicing, and using new recipes to promote flexibility.

- Patient learns how to portion foods for a meal, mini-meal, and/or snack:

  1. using measuring cups and other apparatus
  2. using pre-portioned foods (like a frozen chicken potpie or frozen burritos)
  3. making eyeball estimates
  4. using other simple, visual guides like a fist, palm, 25-cent coin.

- Patient learns how to order and eat at a restaurant:

    1. identifying balanced meal options
    2. making recovery-supported choices aligned with the meal plan (even if they "fake it 'til they make it")
    3. refraining from symptoms and eating appropriate portions during the meal
    4. refraining from symptoms before and after the meal.

- Patient learns how to combine these skills:

    1. making breakfast at home
    2. buying food for balanced snack on the way to work
    3. gathering food (fishing, hunting, berry picking, etc.)
    4. calling in an order for lunch delivery
    5. packing a mini-meal and eating it on schedule at work
    6. moving their body in ways that meet their recovery goals for activity and rest
    7. meeting a friend at a restaurant for dinner
    8. portioning an appropriate amount of food for a snack
    9. if appropriate to their meal plan, buying and consuming supplemental drinks.

- Patient learns alternative ways to release eating-related stress:

    1. coloring (in a coloring book or on plain paper)
    2. listening to music
    3. journaling
    4. practicing yoga
    5. knitting
    6. playing cards or a board game with others
    7. listening to a guided meditation.

As you can see, Structured Eating's process is highly organized—and radically different from how an eating disorder "organizes" food and eating. Conflict between the two—and the radical change we ask patients to make—creates conflict, anxiety, and resistance.

The planning, practice, and thinking people invest in these skills are arduous—a fact we must acknowledge. Practitioners must work to name-and-explain the conflict, help ease the anxiety, and defuse the resistance. Here's a conversation I had with one patient:

THEM: I'm struggling with this. Planning takes so much work, it's like you have to think about it all day long in order to get everything you need—or even one thing you need.

ME: That's true, and I understand how hard it is right now to generate the level of concentration, planning, and eating that your body needs from you right now.

Remember our previous conversation about how the brain and body work? Right now, your brain and body are learning a new skill, while undoing or unsticking an old pattern. Your stress or "tired brain" is evidence you're *experiencing* the brain and body switching to this new way of working together.

THEM: But it's just so exhausting. I don't know if I'm doing it right or will ever learn how to do it right.

ME: OK. Let's talk about something else for a minute: neuroplasticity in infants.

THEM: What?

ME: Hang with me for a second. What does an infant learn by the time she is 24 months old?

THEM: Uh. Well, how to eat solid food, pick up things with its fingers, learn to walk and talk.

ME: That's neuroplasticity at work. At birth, the brain has 100 billion neurons, with about 2,500 synapses each. By age two, there are six times as many: 15,000 synapses per neuron. To create the neural network that lets us learn and remember how to walk and talk, the brain creates hundreds of millions of new synapses. However, if we don't use synapses often enough, the brain prunes them out.

THEM: What, a kid is gonna suddenly stop learning to walk because the brain cuts off some synapses?

ME: No, a kid learns to walk because she *keeps practicing*—that is, falling and getting back up. The practice creates more synapses and strengthens the existing networks.

THEM: OK, I get it. But what *you* don't get is how impossible it is to eat the way you're telling me to.

ME: Well, learning to walk *is* hard, but I grant you that it's not as hard as some other things. Think about how long it took you to learn to read. What things does a kid have to learn, remember, and practice *before* they can read?

THEM: The alphabet and how letters sound.

ME: Yup. They also have to learn and remember which letters have more than one sound (a, c, e, g, i, o, u), and different letters that make the *same* sound (c and k, g and j). Then they learn, apply, and remember word rules—even if the rules don't make much (if any) sense: the A is long when a word ends with a silent E; you say ate instead of eated. It takes time to integrate all these concepts. Remind you of anything?

THEM: I guess you'll say it's like me learning my meal plan.

ME: Right now, you are in the earliest stages of learning how to feed your body what it needs. Structured Eating is like learning the alphabet.

Fortunately, because you're *doing* it, your body *internalizes* the skill by making thousands of synapses. While you learned (or is it learnt?) to read, you didn't feel every new neural pathway. But your skills still advanced from "A, B, D, MNOZ, sing wiff me!" to "I am Sam. Sam I am ... I do not like green eggs and ham" to "It was a dark and stormy night." Integrated Eating follows the same pattern; you will master it by concentrating, learning, making mistakes, and practicing. You're not gonna notice when your brain creates synapses.

THEM: It still sounds exhausting.

ME: I get it. I promise to remind you regularly that, like your reading "teachers," I know you can do this. *The more you practice, the more smoothly the body and brain work together in this new way—and the easier it becomes for you.* I'm going to remind you that Structured Eating's planning, thinking, and choosing are vastly different than what an eating disorder does: fantasizing about eating, villainizing food, shaming your body, attacking you, and so on. Remember that you are giving your body what it needs, right now—and that your body is learning to reciprocate—by making millions of synapses. You will get from the ABCs to Dr. Seuss and beyond.

Remembering to Repeat

Notice how often we said "remember" and "remind" in the conversation above? We cannot say things only once to a person whose eating disorder is assailing them 24/7 with repetitious, destructive messages.

As clinicians and advocates for the person's body, we need to repeat the science, spirit, and experience of recovery. We do this for many reasons— starting with the fact that eating disorders are far more recalcitrant than, say, a seven-year-old who resists doing homework.

Imagine your child getting home from the first day of school. Now imagine saying: "Do your homework, dear," and the child does it flawlessly every day for the rest of the year, without another reminder. Not gonna happen! (By the way, I suspect our kids have an accurate count of how many times this year their father and I "prodded" them about homework.)

When inexperienced at something or still learning how to do it (like bike riding, speaking a new language, or remembering to do homework), we rely on an experienced and knowledgeable person to instruct us—and prod us. The instructors will give us the same instructions and prompts (Did you do your food logs?) over and over, especially at first. Early in the learning curve, we will (especially if we're human) feel frustrated and incompetent. We'll also be skeptical of and resentful toward the instructor.

Over time, of course, we internalize the skills and happily ride our bike all over, speak language *x* fluently, and finish our homework (even if we stay in school for 25 years!). In a perfect world, we would remember and feel grateful for every instructor and send them birthday cards. In the real world, we probably take these skills for granted, forget who taught us, and have little or no memory of exactly how we learned them.

Some people with eating disorders have lost or never learned the essential skill of nourishing their body. Eating disorders can create mental and sensory amnesia around eating. Some people may acknowledge that other parts of their life are disordered, but deny that their eating is out of whack. This may seem impossible or nonsensical if you've never treated people with eating disorders (and, sometimes, even when you've done it for years).

Nevertheless, these realities mean we need repetition to teach recovery skills. We must repeat the instructions to patients, explain the rationales behind the instructions, encourage their practice (another word for repetition), and hold them accountable.

Recovery from an eating disorder is disruptive and disorienting. A clinician's words may be "heard" or hit home in dramatically different ways from one week (or day, or month) to the next. We need to talk about the "same thing" in different ways.

For instance, clinicians and recovered people employ many metaphors for eating disorders (in addition to our earlier list, we've heard: professional actor, aesthete, passive observer, asshole, God, puppeteer). We need to recognize and utilize each moment and metaphor as recovery/teaching/learning opportunities.

Into Real Life

Now, let's see how Structured Eating operates in a patient's day.

Of course, we start with the clinical nutritional goal, depending on the patient's diagnosis and symptoms. We achieve the goals with ratios of essential macronutrients: carbohydrates: protein: fat: fruit and vegetables.

Depending on diagnosis and other factors, the clinical nutritional goals for people in treatment for eating disorders are:

*   Weight restoration: this hypercaloric, nutrient-dense plan meets the body's needs of people with severe weight loss, which leads to electrolyte imbalance, organ failure, and other life-threatening outcomes. The appropriate ratio for meals is 3:2:1:2.
*   Weight maintenance: this plan reflects intrinsic eating; that is, eating in synch with how the body operates. We use it for clients within or moving toward a "safe" weight range, while clients work on purging, bingeing, restricting, chronic dieting, and other symptoms. The appropriate ratio for meals is 2:1:1:1.
*   Metabolic balance: unbalanced/disordered metabolism results from compulsive emotional and/or binge eating, compulsive and/or excessive

exercise, conditions like polycystic ovary syndrome (PCOS), pre-diabetes, diabetes, and other problems. This plan restores metabolic systems while combating eating disorder symptoms. This approach does not focus on changing the patient's body shape or size, the goal is restoring metabolic balance. The appropriate ratio for meals is 1:2:1:2.

Breakfast

During sleep we are much like hibernating bears or the nighttime, set-back furnace. Because we are at rest (and, therefore, not eating), our body shifts into a fasting state that uses less energy *and* consumes each calorie more slowly and more efficiently. The energy we need for life functioning while at rest is called our basal metabolic rate (BMR). During the night, our body also produces hormones to help us fall asleep and stay asleep. Our brains are wired to stop producing those hormones when the sun rises, so we wake up and get going.

Simply opening our eyes and waking from slumber demands more energy units—and requires the body to use them more quickly. This creates a natural "stress" situation in the body, where blood sugar is low, and we need to meet our spiking energy needs within 30–60 minutes. Simultaneously our brain waves shift from the slower theta-delta zone into higher-frequency beta waves associated with alertness and focus. When functioning smoothly, our natural inner environment creates a desire to welcome a mindful morning meal.

However, people with active eating disorders usually don't experience morning as a time of vitality, drive, or even hunger. Instead, morning is a time of stress, anxiety, rushing, and symptomatic eating.

The chorus of eating disorder thoughts, voices, and abuse are major culprits behind a patient's delayed, skipped, chaotic, or compromised breakfast.

One of my younger patients wakes up worried that she will be bullied on the school bus. Immersed in thoughts like "Will they pick on me today?" or "What will I say back?" or "Where will I sit?" her anxiety intensifies while she brushes her teeth and gets dressed. By the time she sits for breakfast, anxiety has consumed her. Now she must deal with food. She demands that her mom not let the foods touch each other on the plate, "or else, I just can't eat it." When she finally does eat, she's nauseous and feels stuffed after only a few bites. And this is just *the first 45 minutes* of living with her eating disorder today.

Morning anxiety is common for people with eating disorders. Anxiety also tends to blunt hunger cues and invite symptom use. One of my patients regularly has "crisis" days with terrible nightmares and morning anxiety attacks. We came up with a safe, easy breakfast we call the "crisis meal." She always has a crisis meal in the house, within easy reach.

Modern-day culture doesn't help much with "starting the day on the right foot." Few of us get up, create space and time to meditate, read the newspaper, quietly pray, set intentions for today, eat a solid meal, or calmly sip a rich cup of coffee *before* moving into the rest of our day. Instead, morning may look more like this.

The alarm clock goes off and our body reacts with a mixture of panic, dread, and exhaustion. Turning off the alarm, we see the "smart" phone flooded with text messages and emails. We may start flipping through social media—even while rushing to get ourselves, our children, our pets, and our computers ready to go out the door. Forget those theta waves, we open our eyes and plunge into hyperarousal. When morning becomes "to-do" management, we're more likely to skip breakfast. Or we delay it until stuck in traffic, mindlessly snarfing a coffee and donut from the drive-through window.

A patient and I discussed a similar scenario recently. She admits that she wakes up early enough to eat breakfast at home and describes her mornings as hectic. Before leaving the house, her usual morning included:

• showering
• getting dressed
• putting on makeup
• gathering everything she needs (or thinks she might need) to be ready for class
• cleaning up her home, because she had to leave it "perfect" before leaving.

I fed back her words.

ME: OK, what I just heard you say is that making your home look "perfect" while nobody's there is more important that feeding your body. If that is true, then we need to understand why. If it's not true, then you have to be willing to change your actions in the morning.

HER: Well, when you say it like that, "no." My body is more important, but it feels hard to eat before I've "produced" a clean apartment.

ME: I understand that, and I'd suggest that the clean apartment may represent or indicate a deeper issue for you and your therapist to work on. Meanwhile, how can we create a way for you to eat a structured breakfast before you leave the house, no matter what else you do in the morning?

HER: I'm not sure. Maybe I could make something the night before and not eat it until the morning.

ME: That's a good idea and very doable. Now let's plan what foods to put in those pre-prepared breakfast meals.

As patients gain more experience with Structured Eating, they will also experience a sense of morning energy that they haven't felt in a long while. This energy is dramatically different from morning rush freneticism. The rewards of nutrition-fueled body energy are enticing for someone who eats chaotically in the morning.

Breakfast Meal Structure

Like the other Structured Eating *meals,* breakfast contains foods from all four essential macronutrients categories: complex carbohydrates, protein, fat, fruit/vegetable.

We build the structured meal plan to meet the patient's current diagnostic and clinical needs. In every case, we explain the rationale for ratios and portions.

We find that patients manage balanced eating more successfully when we make it less complicated, more structured, easier to remember, and easier to repeat. Our structure is not rigid or monotonous. But it does "short-circuit" the eating disorder's chaotic, often paralyzing reactions to a never-ending list of options.

The practice helps lessen patients' stress, thinking, or obsessing about food while they prepare a meal and eat it. In addition, we help reduce patient (and eating disorder) resistance by providing concrete recovery-focused choices in structured meal plans.

For instance, a patient says: "I usually eat oatmeal for breakfast." I respond:

> OK, great. Let's start with your oatmeal and explore how it serves your body and your needs. Oatmeal is a complex carbohydrate, so you have that covered. It doesn't have all the ingredients for a balanced meal, so oatmeal alone is incomplete. Oatmeal has fiber in it, which may leave you feeling full. But, because it's not balanced, oatmeal does not leave you *fed*—as in, giving your body what it needs right now.
>
> Let's think about types of protein we can add. I've got a list of easy-to-make protein/fat combination foods like eggs, cheese, nuts, nut butters, and dairy with milk fat. Protein and fat balance your blood sugar and maintain your energy for more than an hour. Let's choose how to put them together.

This approach immediately shifts the conversation away from *worrying about* fat and calories to *looking for* foods that build a balanced meal. It also diminishes fears about whether there are too many or too few items on the plate.

Most of our patients can switch from leery to looking—at least for long enough to make the food choices. Once they've chosen a protein/fat combination to add to the oatmeal we look for a fruit or veg (like banana or celery). In a matter of moments, their way-more-balanced-breakfast (say, oatmeal with nuts and raisins) is simple to visualize, make, and eat in the same bowl. Many folks proudly share their clever "one-bowl miracle" with others.

Of course, not all balanced breakfasts are alike (or need to be alike). There is some variation in how people's bodies break down food combinations. Let's take someone with breakfast meal plan options of cereal with nuts, banana, and milk on Monday and peanut butter and jelly sandwich and apple on Tuesday. On Monday, they were hungry sooner than on Tuesday. That's not bad news; we just note the information.

After regularly eating yogurt, granola, and fruit for breakfast, one of my patients said this combination wasn't working now that she's pregnant. I suggested an egg sandwich and piece of fruit instead. A few days later, she reported back her sense that, for now, the new combo was a better balance for her body. With that understanding and exploration, we came up with two other higher-protein options for her breakfasts. (Noticing is welcome recovery progress whenever it happens and it builds skills for the Mindful Eating phase.)

Making It Real: Meal Plans and Food Logs

During Structured Eating, patients and providers need meal plans and food logs to shape and track progress. They help all of us to home in on the crucial recovery skills of when, what, and how much to eat.

Meal Plans

The meal plan gives patients firm guidance and direction for when and what to eat. The sample meal plan shown in Table 3.1 is for breakfast. The framework is intentionally simple, specific, and directive:

- row one: the clinical goal and associated ratio of essential macronutrients (carbohydrates: protein: fat: fruit/vegetable)
- remaining rows: examples of three different breakfast meals that meet the clinical goal.

Food Logs

We don't use Structured Eating food logs to obsess over portions, calories, and so on (Table 3.2). Instead, the patient "checks off" items to collect data for themselves and their clinicians.

For each eating event, the patient tracks:

- time of day (the breakfast log also asks the patient to note when they woke up)
- eating event designation (meal, mini-meal, snack)

- food consumed
- carbohydrates (C), protein (P), fat (F), fruit/vegetable (F/V)

  - O = over; ate more than plan
  - A = ate adequate for the plan
  - U = under; ate less than the plan

- activity/exercise/movement (how I moved my body before, during, or after the eating event)
- eating disorder symptoms I used
- recovery goal (for next day part or eating event).

Table 3.1 Meal Plan: Breakfast

	Weight Restoration *3:2:1:2*	*Weight Maintenance* *2:1:1:1*	*Metabolic Balance* *1:2:1:2*
Breakfast 1	2-egg omelette with 1 slice of cheese, spinach, and mushroom. 1½ cup home fries, mixed fruit cup	1 egg with 1 slice of cheese, spinach, and mushroom. 1 cup home fries	2-egg omelette with a slice of cheese, spinach, and mushroom. ½ cup home fries, mixed fruit cup
Breakfast 2	1½ cup 2% Greek-style yogurt with ¾ cup of granola, ¼ cup of chopped nuts, 1½ cups of frozen berries	1 cup 2% Greek-style yogurt with ½ cup of granola, ¼ cup of chopped nuts, ¾ cup of frozen berries	1½ cup 2% Greek-style yogurt with ¼ cup of granola, ¼ cup of chopped nuts, 1½ cups of frozen berries
Breakfast 3	2 toaster waffles with 2 Tbs peanut butter, 1 banana, 2 tsp butter, 2 Tbs syrup, with 2 Tbs wheat germ sprinkled on top. Glass of milk	2 toaster waffles with 2 Tbs peanut butter, 1 banana, 2 tsp butter	1 toaster waffle with 2 Tbs peanut butter, 1 banana, 2 tsp butter. Glass of milk

Modern food log technologies provide multiple ways for clinician and client to reinforce the organization and practice of "doing" Structured Eating. Clients use food logs for support and accountability. Clinicians use them to see what, when, and how much clients are eating. The detail and context illustrate the story of the client's day and provide valuable data to discuss when we next meet in person.

Table 3.2 Food Log: Breakfast

Goal	Wake Up	Time	Eating Event	Food Consumed	C	P	F	F/V	Activity/ Exercise/ Movement	Symptoms	Recovery Goal
Weight restoration	6:30 am	07:30	Breakfast	2 eggs, 1 piece of toast, 1 container of yogurt, 3 cups of berries	U	A	U	O	Walked to work 20 blocks	Restrict	Work on volume, eating low-calorie, high-fiber foods to feel full
Weight maintenance	5:15 am	7:45 am	Bfast	½ cup fat-free cottage cheese, 2 toaster waffles, 1 cup berries	A	A	U	A	Run 5:45 am 3 miles		Eat within first hour of waking up. Plan early-morning snack on early-morning run days. Stop buying fat-free diary products
Metabolic balance	07:45	8:10 am	Brekkie	Bacon, egg, and cheese on bagel	O	A	A	U	Yoga class at 9:30		Do another yoga class next week! Do this breakfast again with English muffin instead of bagel and add tomato

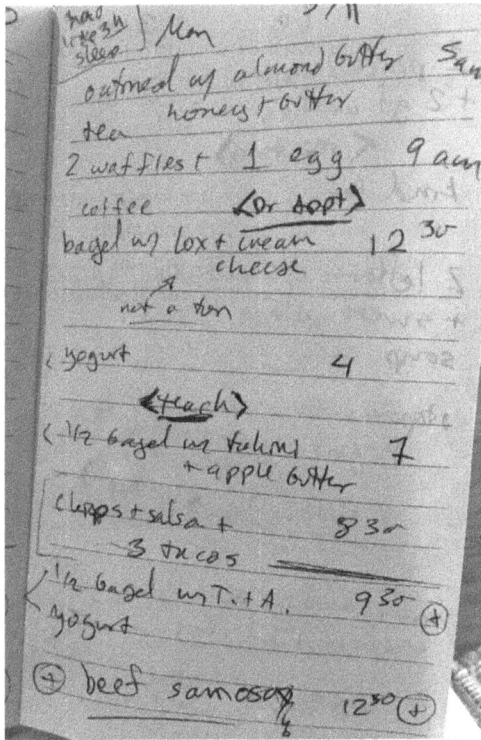

Figure 3.1 Handwritten food log which the patient emailed to his provider.

Email

A client on a metabolic balance plan emails me when and what he ate for breakfast (Figure 3.1):

> Bacon, egg, and cheese on bagel

I replied:

> This is a great effort. Next time you eat this, try it on an English muffin with tomato and choose either cheese or bacon.

Text

A client with compulsive eating symptoms is working on combining a rotating three plan with well-defined times between eating events. She texts me "before" and "after" photos of her meal. I can see the selections and portions clearly. I also see that she didn't meet our meal-spacing goal.

I replied:

> You're right on point with your portions and we need to honor your timing goals for the rest of the day.

Phone App

A client struggling with restriction sends her logs via an application platform (like Recovery Record). The app gathers and shares a detailed account of eating events with clinician and client. The app stamps the time (key info for us) and invites the client to add comments and observations (Figure 3.2).

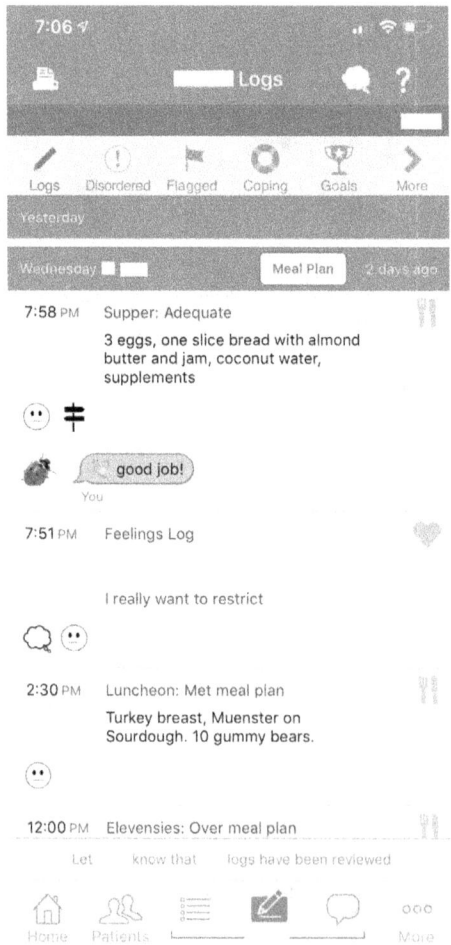

Figure 3.2 Food log app completed by patient and emailed to her provider.

I texted and asked her to eat three specific foods when she got home. She followed those instructions, let me know, and I replied: Good job!

Computers and Tablets

A client working on binge and purge cycles uploads and fills in our food log on their tablet. When we meet, we go over each eating event. I give specific suggestions to strengthen our strategy for reaching the clinical goal:

> Hey, this Tuesday breakfast is great. You have two complex carbs, a protein, and fruit. I see you have fat-free yogurt here. Remember how and why your body needs and uses fat. This week let's use 2% yogurt and add some nuts.

The "Cloud"

Clients can share food logs as "cloud" files, stored on the Internet. We can add responses within those files (Google Docs or Google Sheets, documents or spreadsheets saved to Microsoft's OneDrive or Apple's iCloud, etc.) or email our responses.

One of my clients uses PowerPoint to create daily food logs with text, images, drawings, and other imaginative elements. Who knew that the food log could be a medium for recovery-oriented art? In fact, clients can use almost any mundane element of treatment to invent "unexpected" creativity.

Paper

And, yes, some people really do print out and fill in *paper versions* of our food log for us to discuss during sessions. The 10,000-year-old technology of pencil and paper still works!

We also have a patient who sends us photos of the Post-It notes she uses to log.

Morning Snack

It's common for our patients to resist the morning snack. No matter the diagnosis or symptomatology, people with eating disorders must contend with anxiety, blunted cues, rebellion, fear, intrusive thoughts, and/or body image shame. Because eating disorders fire away all day, the first snack tends to get a blast of: "*No way* I'm doing this!"

When a patient adamantly says no to eating, we can pique their interest with metabolism information—even if that interest originates in eating disorder obsessions. I usually break out one of my MMTs: *mighty metabolism talks*. I always start with: "The facts and functions of the body's metabolism are immutable." In one of my MMTs, I ask clients to picture being on a camping trip.

The wellbeing (and survival) of you and your fellow campers depend on the *campfire*'s warmth—ergo, *the fire must stay lit.* If you add a few logs before bedtime, the fire will burn overnight, and leave only a few embers in the morning.

When you wake up to embers, you have choices:

1. Do nothing, and your fire will burn out completely.
2. Feed the fire with small twigs, and your fire will flare up briefly, then quickly return to embers, no matter how much you stoke it.
3. Pile large and/or wet logs on the embers; the fire will sputter unevenly and soon go out.
4. Add dry, moderate-sized logs *at a consistent pace throughout the day*, and your fire will keep you warm all day—and burn into the night.

It's the same with your body and food. After waking up with energy "embers," you have choices:

1. Skip or delay adding food to your energy-using body, and the energy fire burns out.
2. Randomly eat tiny "twig" amounts of food throughout the day and your energy flares up briefly, then quickly return to embers, no matter how many quick-burning "twig" foods you eat.
3. Sporadically or continually eat unbalanced foods (like the large, wet logs) throughout the day and your fire will sputter unevenly and eventually go out.
4. Eat a balanced meal and snacks *at a consistent pace throughout the day*, and your body's early-morning energy embers become a steady, efficient fire to keep you stable, safe, and productive all day.

In nearly all conversations, clinicians must also work to differentiate the eating disorder "voice" from the recovery "voice." The eating disorder conjures up excuses, irrational arguments, and obsessive thoughts to facilitate decisions and actions that benefit the disorder, instead of the person. It says things like:

*   I'm not hungry, so I can skip morning snack.
*   I need way more than this puny snack, or else I'll starve.
*   I'm too rushed this morning; I'll raid the candy jar at work or eat a bigger lunch.

The recovery "voice" says things like:

*   I may not be hungry for a snack, but I have this trail mix, so I'll eat it.
*   I'm afraid I'll starve if I don't eat something more than this trail mix, but, right now, I'll trust my meal plan.
*   I'm in a rush so I'll get an egg sandwich with my morning coffee.

Depending on the patient's needs and/or life situation, they will need two or three floating snacks. As with other eating events, we aim for simple. Most folks have peanut butter or cheese at home. Both are versatile in balanced snacks. You can spread peanut butter or add cheese to many things (bread, apples, rice cakes, crackers, etc.) and you have a balanced and sufficient snack. (See Chapter 4 for afternoon and evening snack meal plans.)

Remember that snacks must include a food with *both* protein and fat, paired with a macronutrient of fruit, vegetable, or complex carbohydrate:

- protein and fat + fruit
- protein and fat + vegetable
- protein and fat + complex carbohydrate.

And we make it simple for our patients to remember by the designations of 2:2, 2:1, or 1:1 (Tables 3.3 and 3.4).

Table 3.3 Meal Plan: Morning Snack

	Weight Restoration 2:2	*Weight Maintenance* 2:1	*Metabolic Balance* 1:1
Morning snack 1	1 cup 2% yogurt, ⅔ cup granola	1 cup 2% yogurt, ⅓ cup granola	½ cup 2% yogurt, ⅓ cup granola
Morning snack 2	½ cup trail mix, Boost supplement	½ cup trail mix	¼ cup trail mix
Morning snack 3	2 Tbs almond butter, 1 apple, 1 small box of raisins	2 Tbs almond butter, apple	1 Tbs almond butter, apple

It's Not Even Noon Yet!

We're less than halfway through the day and we've covered a ton of detail already. Now, imagine operating with an eating-disordered, malnourished body and brain ... while *also* trying to:

- understand the information and strategies in this chapter (and the next chapter)
- use the information and strategies in this chapter (and the next chapter)
- trust that it all will nourish you.

Table 3.4 Food Log: Morning Snack

Goal	Time	Eating Event	Food Consumed	C	P	F	F/V	Activity/ Exercise/ Movement	Symptoms	Recovery Goal
Weight restoration	10:30 am	Snack	Apple	NA	U	U	A	-	Restrict	Follow my meal plan
Weight maintenance	5:00 am	Early-morning snack	Clif Bar	A	A	A	-	Run 6 miles	Over-exercise	Do not run over 3 miles on Wednesday
Metabolic balance	11:00 am	Morning snack	1 Tbs peanut butter, banana, 4 large handfuls of m&ms from candy jar, 2 handfuls of trail mix from snack room, 2 more Tbs peanut butter at my desk	O	O	O	A		Compulsive eating/binge	Get back on track for next meal

During Structured Eating, we help patients develop their "what to do next" strategies. We invite them to consider doing the next right thing—in this next moment. Sounds simple but isn't easy. It takes daily practice—and helps build the skills they need to transition into Mindful Eating.

- If I eat a balanced meal or snack, the right next step is to do it again in another few hours.
- If I skip or delay eating, the right next step is to eat *now*.
- If I've eaten in a symptomatic manner, the right next step is to journal, reach out for support, and/or check my meal plan to know when to eat again.
- If I'm having eating disorder-related thoughts, the right next step is to not act on the thought and then eat what is on my meal plan.

The right next step is always in alignment with recovery, no matter what it is!

Just one reason why recovery is hard work.

Bibliography

Geisel, T. *Green Eggs and Ham* (New York: Random House, 1960).

L'Engle, M. *A Wrinkle in Time* (New York: Farrar, Straus and Giroux, 1962).

Reis, H.T., Collins, W.A., and Berscheid, E. (2000). The relationship context of human behavior and development. *Psychological Bulletin*, 126(6), 844–872.

4 Structured Eating in Real Life
After Noon

Throughout Structured Eating, we reinforce a recovery truth for our patients: your first priority is eating, so that your body will ride the waves of its daily energy tides, generate the energy it needs, and nurture your healing.

Midday Tension

If a client's fuel and metabolism haven't kept pace with circadian rhythms (Figure 4.1) and energy needs during the morning, midday is a big problem. An adequate, balanced breakfast and snack supply enough fuel for a patient's body to *reach* midday. What happens next is up to the food decisions they make.

The most common point of resistance at lunch time is "I can't handle my stress without my symptoms." Therefore, we need multiple techniques to help our clients through this time of day. To bring structured eating successfully into the patient's work/school/home day, patient and nutritionist must formulate balanced meals that work "in real life."

For example, lunch—and other eating events—are challenging for patients with fluctuating and/or unpredictable schedules. People struggling with eating disorders already have difficulty with boundaries. Carving out mealtimes feels nearly impossible if they are at home raising children, working multiple jobs, going to school, have rotating work shifts, are working from home, are unemployed or underemployed, or doing several of these things at once! These folks often use a "snacky lunch" habit to get by: grabbing a donut, drive-thru McDonald's burger, ramen noodles, "nutrition" bar, or three bowls of cereal to compensate for a missed midday meal.

One of my patients sometimes senses her first hunger signal around 11:30 am, but she reports: "Work stress and meetings that run into (or through) lunch time *prohibit* me from paying attention to these signals." For her, setting a "time to eat" alarm is a simple and practical Structured Eating strategy.

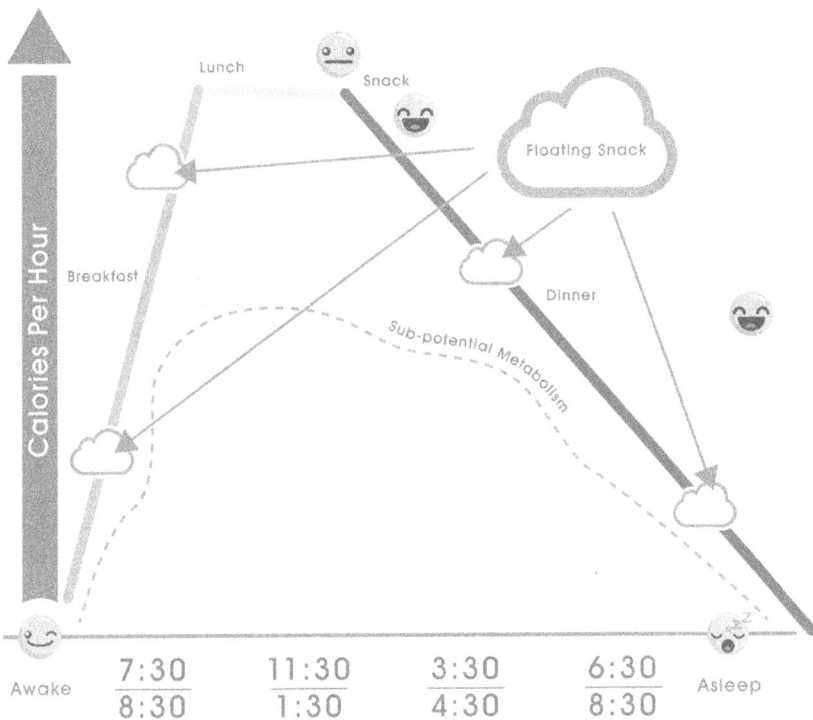

Figure 4.1 Circadian rhythms.

People with eating disorders may feel guilty about eating balanced lunch foods (turkey sandwich and pickle vs. oatmeal). I'm reminded of a patient whose lunch choices alternate between nothing and small items (granola bar and/or three dried banana pieces).

We developed simple, workable strategies. She bought easy-to-assemble lunch foods like peanut butter, hummus, bread, soup, apple sauce, and cheese to the break room refrigerator at work. For the days she's off site making sales calls, we made a list of places to stop for meals to eat there or take out and eat elsewhere. She also kept microwavable meals in her freezer for days she worked from home.

But our work doesn't simply stop with identifying viable lunches. I believe that purging, bingeing, restricting, and other symptoms are *all* signs of body, mind, and spirit deprivation.

Stepping into Deprivation

We do our patients an injustice when we sidestep the call to collaborate with colleagues and explore clients' deeper life deprivations. These deprivations engender distortive eating disorder thoughts that fuel symptom behavior every day.

For instance, the changes we ask people to make may ignite embodied shame that erupts whenever they do anything *other than* numb and/or deprive themselves. Self-nurturing behavior often feels antithetical to the shame-based belief that "I am *unworthy of any nurture*." This shame frequently results from trauma (sexual, mental, physical, emotional abuse; racism; poverty; addiction; addicted loved ones; abandonment, etc.) people endured in the past—and may still endure today.

Processing shame is a much taller order than developing, following, and repeating meal plans. So, dietitians (and other providers) must work in multiple dimensions, even during the concrete phase of Structured Eating. We must collaborate with treatment teams to tackle these and other recovery-related challenges that our patients face.

While our patients work on issues which invited the eating disorder in, we must align our nutrition approach and language with the patient's situation right now—whether it's a recent divorce, mood or personality disorder, obsessive-compulsive disorder, grief, and so on. This may mean rethinking how we respond to deprivation-driven symptoms. For instance, I no longer use phrases like "you have to eat a balanced meal." I've learned to move toward language like this:

> I understand that eating this way is hard.
>
> I understand that eating like this brings up feelings that you are not worthy of nourishment, serenity, meaning, or love in your life.
>
> Together we can change that. That change is difficult and sometimes draining, and you don't have to do it alone.
>
> Together, we will challenge some of the old and familiar stories with new actions.
>
> The actions include eating with structure and on a schedule. Eating like that rebels against the old, familiar eating disorder stories—which are really myths. Eating like that has as much impact (or more) as any mantras, affirmations, or promises you make to yourself or other people.
>
> Eating with structure and on a schedule may feel wrong. It will go against everything you know right now.
>
> But it will not always feel like this. And I promise to hold hope for you, even during times you think you can't possibly hold on to hope or don't deserve anything better than your illness(es).

Remember: eating is fear-filled and difficult for people with eating disorders. Their safety is in our hands and the hands of our colleagues. Together, we must teach them tools for safe and simple eating and living.

Lunch

Thanks to circadian rhythms, our body reaches its highest metabolism and energy usage of the day in the middle of the day. Now, the body needs a fresh package of balanced nutrients to keep blood sugar steady and metabolism running efficiently for the next part of the day.

When a patient goes off their lunch meal plan, their body can't keep up with its midday energy demands. That brings on sluggishness, difficulty concentrating, fatigue, and so forth—while increasing the potential for symptomatic behaviors and *additional* problematic food decisions.

Structured Eating's science-based approach helps address the chronic eating disorder complaint: "I don't have time for lunch." For instance, we describe how and why our bodies evolved to (literally) "make hay while the sun shines." Around midday, the body revs up to metabolize and consume energy at higher rates. Brains are awake and alert (in the alpha- and beta-wave range) throughout the daytime hours. So, we discuss the relevant implications:

- Your body needs today's lunch "fuel" to maintain a steady energy flow that keeps your brain awake and alert for the next few hours.
- In your life situation (work, school, child rearing, etc.) you are likely to be busy during midday.
  - Busyness can distract us from the body's cueing system of hunger and satiety.
  - Distraction makes it easier for eating disorder symptoms to surface.
  - Busyness and distraction shift your brain waves and nervous system into anxious, compulsive, and/or obsessive mode.

When naturally occurring midday hunger sensations coincide with an activated sympathetic nervous system (SNS), emotions become especially intense and fraught.

On a busy day, you and I may experience an SNS high when bouncing from one thing to another. However, many people with eating disorder experience SNS activation repeatedly every day. Plus, their frequent SNS activation stresses the brain and other organs in a malnourished body already holding anxiety, trauma, or depression!

The eating disorder can "use" SNS episodes to reinforce beliefs such as:

- I'm can't get through this stress without eating comfort food all afternoon.
- I'm in high gear and restricting will keep me there.
- If I feel stressed after lunch, I'll purge to relieve it.

In addition, many people with eating disorders are perfectionistic and deeply involved (emotionally and mentally) in their jobs, classes, and other daily events. This pattern leaves them emotionally and mentally exhausted and/or charged during the day.

Accumulated midday tension creates more vulnerability to "managing" emotions with symptoms like bingeing, purging, restriction, or compulsive eating. When aspects of the day feel overwhelming or out of control, eating behavior is the one thing they can control.

No wonder noontime amplifies patient fear of lunch and its aftermath. Less-than-optimal midday functioning is normal for an eating disorder, and difficult to disrupt. Bottom line: early in treatment, eating structure is essential for people with eating disorders.

Discussing the science of energy conservation can give clinicians a less-fraught path to address lunch-and-beyond fears. Stable, efficient energy use may not be a prime motivation for our clients, but it is important information to have.

A light touch can help patients feel more receptive to the science behind the body at midday.

I sometimes tell patients: "To lunch or not to lunch? That is the question!"

- When you eat a balanced lunch, your body has enough fuel for its higher energy rate.
- If you skip lunch, your body is stuck with only enough fuel for "morning" rates. It quickly falls behind while straining to work at midday rates.
- As the afternoon and its new energy needs progress, your body regresses, steadily losing ground without more balanced fuel.

Here's an illustrative conversation from our practice:

THEM: Lunch is so hard.

REGISTERED DIETITIAN (RD): Tell me more.

THEM: I hate it, because eating lunch is a hassle. It's much easier when I just graze and snarf all day until I go to bed.

RD: Do you remember our conversation last week about circadian rhythms and your body's energy needs around noon? And what happens when the needs don't get met?

THEM: Yes.

RD: So, let me ask you: did you feel tired or irritable yesterday afternoon? Or have trouble concentrating?

THEM: Yeah, I guess so.

RD: That's how our bodies react when we don't give them the kind of fuel they need around lunchtime and later in the afternoon, right?

THEM: If you say so.

RD: Do you think your body did that yesterday?

THEM: Yeah, I guess so. But that's not the only problem with lunch.

RD: Tell me more.

THEM: It sucks trying to figure out when to eat and what to eat.

RD: OK, what time do you wake up?

THEM: 7:00.

RD: And what time do you eat breakfast?

THEM: 8:00.

RD: OK, where are you at noon?

THEM: Most of the time, I'm in a meeting.

RD: OK, let's strategize about the days with meetings over the noon hour. Let's look at your calendar and agree on when you *can* eat lunch?

THEM: Well, those meetings usually end by 1:00, but I avoid going out to lunch with people because it's embarrassing. So, let's say 1:15.

RD: Good. That'll work. Now, let's tackle what to eat. You'll either need to make lunch and bring it to work or grab lunch on your way to work.

THEM: What do I bring or get?

RD: What can you make the night before to bring?

THEM: I always seem to have leftovers. I guess it's easy to pack them.

RD: OK, try that. How about picking something up in the morning?

THEM: Well, I guess I can buy a wrap at the place I get my coffee.

RD: Great, you have two plans to try next week for lunch—and for holding off your afternoon fatigue and irritation.

Lunch Meal Plans

Since lunch is a "full" meal, the meal plan has the same *ratios* as breakfast. Table 4.1 gives three Structured Eating balanced lunch examples for each nutritional goal.

Table 4.1 Meal Plan: Lunch

	Weight Restoration 3:2:1:2	*Weight Maintenance* 2:1:1:1	*Metabolic Balance* 1:2:1:2
Lunch 1	Sandwich on 2 pieces of bread made with 1 cup of tuna salad (2 Tbs mayo), orange, serving of goldfish crackers, 4 oz lemonade	Sandwich on 2 pieces of bread made with ½ cup of tuna salad (2 Tbs mayo), orange	Open-face sandwich on a piece of bread made with 1 cup of tuna salad (2 Tbs mayo), orange, and cup of baby carrots
Lunch 2	Leftovers: 6 oz of chicken breast, 3 cups of penne pasta, 2 cups of broccoli florets, 2 tsp olive oil	Leftovers: 3 oz of chicken breast, 2 cups of penne pasta, 1 cup of broccoli florets, 2 tsp olive oil	Leftovers: 6 oz of chicken breast, 1 cup of penne pasta, 2 cups of broccoli florets, 2 tsp olive oil
Lunch 3	2 slices of cheese pizza, large Greek salad with grilled chicken, serving of croutons, 2 Tbs dressing	2 slices of cheese pizza, small Greek salad with grilled chicken, 2 Tbs dressing	1 slice of cheese pizza, large Greek salad with grilled chicken, 2 Tbs dressing

Lunch Food Logs

As with other eating events, here is a visual representation of the data people gather through their food logs (Table 4.2). Remember, for each eating event, the patient tracks:

- time of day
- food consumed
- eating event designation (meal, mini-meal, snack)
- carbohydrates (C), protein (P), fat (F), fruit/vegetable (F/V)

  - O = over; ate more than plan
  - A = ate adequate for the plan
  - U = under; ate less than the plan

- How I moved my body (before, during, or after the eating event)
- Eating disorder symptoms I used
- Recovery goal (for next day part or eating event).

The Mini-Meal

Our clinical experience indicates that patients do better when the mid-afternoon eating event is more substantial than a snack. I jokingly ask my clients to elect me President of Food,[1] so I can officially establish a mandatory, worldwide *mini-meal*. Luckily, there is no President of Food, *and* we officially made mini-meals part of Integrated Eating.

Larger afternoon eating events are not a new concept. In the 1840s, the British started serving afternoon "tea" (featuring finger-food cucumber, curried chicken, or egg salad sandwiches; bread and jam; little cakes, and so on).

Here's the science behind the mini-meal: when we eat a solid breakfast, morning snack, and lunch, our body's circadian rhythms, energy usage, and brain waves are either on the upswing or at a plateau.

Around mid-afternoon, we hit the "three o'clock slump." Serotonin levels and blood sugar dip, brain waves slow slightly, and metabolic functions start downshifting slowly in preparation for bedtime.

It's easy to find evidence of this universal metabolic shift. Kids need naps. Adults seek caffeine-delivery systems and sweets. Even when the body systems change is gradual, it can feel drastic in the body:

- mental fog
- depressed or low-energy feeling
- fatigue or sleepiness
- physiologic hunger

Table 4.2 Food Log: Lunch

Goal	Time	Eating Event	Food Consumed	C	P	F	F/V	Activity/Exercise/ Movement	Symptoms	Recovery Goal
Weight restoration	12:15	Lunch	Slice of pizza (left the crust), cherry Italian ice	U	U	U	U	Walk 40 blocks	Restrict, compulsive exercise	Eat 100%
Weight maintenance	01:30	Lunch	Ham and cheese on a club roll with lettuce and tomato, bag of pretzels, 2 cupcakes	O	A	O	A		Purge	Eat a larger mini-meal
Metabolic balance	02:45	Late lunch	Chipotle salad bowl with chicken, lettuce, tomato, cheese, taco shell, asked for extra guaca-mole and double chicken	A	A	O	A			Next time choose guac or cheese with this lunch

- craving sugar
- irritability
- difficulty concentrating.

Mid-afternoon is rife with complications and pitfalls for people with eating disorders, depression, and anxiety. Lowered blood sugar and slowing body rhythms create emotional and chemical instability, problematic thought patterns, and symptom use.

We remind our clients that mental and emotional signals are *real* cues from the body: "Poor concentration or fatigue in the afternoon are your body's way of getting your attention to say it needs energy. You need to take these cues seriously and listen."

Like the rest of us, our patients live in everyday environments that encourage cravings. Workplace "snack rooms," campus "snack bars," hallway vending machines, and the kitchen cookie jar overflow with sweet or savory quick-eat foods. It's easy to develop "afternoon is junk food time" habits—and fears.

We make clear to every patient that that sweets and snacking:

- are not bad or inherently wrong
- do not serve our body's afternoon energy and metabolism needs.

Nevertheless, people in our care often tell themselves (and us, if we're lucky): "Oh no, I'm not hungry for anything right now" or "I'm too hungry and the candy is right here."

Our battle cry is: the mini-meal is not optional. It's essential—and can literally save the day. Eating the mini-meal is your responsibility to your body. Restricting and sweets can't do the job.

Because "something is better than nothing," we frequently use the "placeholder" strategy to address resistance to mini-meals.

For example, a patient only eats crackers for her mini-meal. We explain why lentil soup, crackers, and string cheese make a more balanced and adequate choice for her energy needs. She doesn't bite. So, we say: "For the time being, the crackers and string cheese will be our temporary placeholder until you can tolerate more. You might struggle to eat the string cheese, but it will be easier than eating the lentil soup."

We also encourage patients to see the mini-meal as a *treat* that propels us through the afternoon "slump." In Structured Eating, "treat" is not defined as foods we compulsively crave; those eating events are rarely balanced. Instead, mini-meal's "treat" is the wonderful, rewarding nutrition that gives our body what it needs at an important time of our day.

To review, the mini-meal has the same macronutrients as a meal, but smaller portions:

- complex carbohydrate
- protein
- fat
- fruit or vegetable.

The ratios are weight restoration 2:1:1:1, weight maintenance 1:1:1:1, and metabolic balance 0.5:1:1:1 (Table 4.3).

Mini-Meal Meal Plans

We don't overdo the meal plan conversation every week; we discuss it once or twice and then refer to it when needed. No matter the meal plan, we continually give our patients concrete and realistic options for completing it.

Table 4.3 Meal Plan: Mini Meal

	Weight Restoration 2:1:1:1	*Weight Maintenance 1:1:1:1*	*Metabolic Balance 0.5:1:1:1*
Mini meal 1	2 servings of crackers, 1 Kraft Singles–sized square of cheese, 1 cup grapes	1 serving of crackers, 1 Kraft Singles–sized square of cheese, 1 cup grapes	½ serving of crackers, 1 Kraft Singles–sized square of cheese, 1 cup grapes
Mini meal 2	3 rice cakes with ½ cup egg salad, 6 pieces of celery	2 rice cakes with ½ cup egg salad, 6 pieces of celery	1 rice cake with ½ cup egg salad, 6 pieces of celery
Mini meal 3	2 medium tortilla wraps with 2 Tbs cashew butter, small box raisins	1 medium tortilla wrap with 2 Tbs cashew butter, small box of raisins	1 small tortilla wrap with 2 Tbs cashew butter, small box of raisins

Here's a resistance response conversation with an at-home parent about mini-meals:

THEM: I just don't have time or a place to make or eat a mini-meal.

RD: Where are you most days around 3:00 pm?

THEM: Running errands before getting the kids at school.

RD: What foods do you usually have around the house?

THEM: I'm not sure. And every time I look in my fridge, I think: "I have nothing to eat!"

RD: Do you have eggs? Cheese? Hummus? Soup? Canned tuna? Peanut butter?

THEM: I have eggs and cheese and a jar of peanut butter. I don't like hummus!

RD: Do you have bread or crackers or other carbs?

THEM: Yes, I have a box of Triscuits and a box of frozen waffles. I also have individual bags of pretzels hanging around.

RD: What about carrots or fruit?

THEM: I have baby carrots and some diced pineapple in cans.

RD: Sounds like you can make yourself a mini-meal of two slices of cheese on Triscuits with those baby carrots on the side for today. Tomorrow, use a toaster waffle with peanut butter and the can of pineapple. How does that sound?

THEM: Well, I guess I could do that if I'm home. I'll probably be shopping before picking up the kids from school on Thursday.

RD: OK. Think about where you'll be driving Thursday. On or near your route, where is the closest (café, bodega, grocery store)?

THEM: Well, there's a 7–11 on Kinderkamack Road.

RD: What time can you stop there and get a package of crackers with cheese, and buy a banana, too?

THEM: Around 2:30, I guess, between going to the Stop and Shop and getting the kids.

RD: OK. Let's do that, and then use your food log to show me how it pans out.

Mini-Meal Food Logs (see Table 4.4)

Early-Evening Snack

As we discussed earlier, scheduling the "floating" snack depends on the person's life situation. After the mini meal, they may need to eat a balanced snack:

- a few hours before dinner, when dinner will be on the *late* side (early-evening snack)
- a few hours after dinner, when dinner will be on the *early* side (late-evening snack).

One of my patients with compulsive eating struggles with anxiety and depression along with their eating disorder. They have no problem with balanced eating events through mid-afternoon. The struggles begin an hour or two after the mini-meal. They work late and their workload picks up after 4:30. The combination of stress, anxiety, mental fogginess, depression, and fading blood sugar creates a perfect storm for compulsive eating.

For example, they frequently interpret mental fogginess *as hunger* late in the afternoon. Eating sweets gives them a temporary jolt of energy, but

Table 4.4 Food Log: Mini Meal

Goal	Time	Eating Event	Food Consumed	C	P	F	F/V	Activity/ Exercise/ Movement	Symptoms	Recovery Goal
Weight restoration	4:30 pm	Mini-meal	2 hard-boiled eggs, Nutrigrain bar, apple	U	O	U	A		Restrictive	Add carbs in next snack
Weight maintenance	3:15 pm	Mini-meal	Protein bar	A	A	A	U		Bad body image distortion all afternoon	Do not let bad body image affect my eating
Metabolic balance	3:55 pm	Mini-meal	Had a cheese stick between meetings	U	A	A	U		Restrictive	Plan next snack no later than 5 pm

the ensuing crash leaves them even more sluggish. It's been a recurring vicious cycle for years.

Together, we created a snack meal plan with what they called "middle-ground choices" to provide nutrients and help stay on track throughout the day. They chose berries instead of candy, and trail mix (with small chunks of chocolate) instead of chocolate-flavored, sweetened yogurt. Instead of the old go-to sweets, they're eating foods that:

- they "like but don't love"
- still give some sense of satisfaction, without overloading the brain's reward center with nanosecond bursts of pleasure
- meet their body's energy needs.

The early-evening snack provides the body with stable influx of energy between mini-meal and dinner. The late-evening snack meets the body's nutritional needs between dinner and bedtime.

In general, we use the early-evening snack when there are two to three hours between mini-meal and dinner. We use the late-evening snack when there are two to three hours between dinner and bedtime.

One of my restrictive patients was eating dinner early, and then "snacking" on a few mixed nuts later on. She argued that the snack worked fine because it came a few hours after dinner. When we dove into the details, she was hungry for more before bed, but "snacking" allowed her to feel like she ate enough. Except that it wasn't. I gave her my "a balanced snack is not the same as snacking" talk and encouraged her to eat the snack portions in her meal plan. At the next session, she reported eating a full portion and feeling more fed before bed—a concrete step toward greater understanding of the meal plan's rationale and outcomes.

Remember that snacks must include a food with *both* protein and fat, paired with a macronutrient of fruit, vegetable, or complex carbohydrate, and the ratios are 2:2, 2:1 and 1:1 (Tables 4.5 and 4.6).

Pre-Dinner Snack Meal Plans and Food Logs

Table 4.5 Meal Plan: Afternoon Snack

	Weight Restoration 2:2	Weight Maintenance 2:1	Metabolic Balance 1:1
Afternoon snack 1	2 serving of crackers, 1/4 cup hummus	1 serving of cracker, 1/4 cup hummus	1 serving of crackers, 2 Tbs hummus
Afternoon snack 2	1 large apple, 2 cheese rounds	1 small apple, 2 cheese rounds	1 small apple, 1 cheese round
Afternoon snack 3	4 pieces of turkey or beef jerky, 1 cup jicama	4 pieces of turkey or beef jerky, 1/2 cup jicama	2 pieces of turkey or beef jerky, ½ cup jicama

Early-Evening Snack Food Logs

Table 4.6 Food Log: Afternoon Snack

Goal	Time	Eating Experience	Food Consumed	C	P	F	F/V	Activity/Exercise/ Movement	Symptoms	Recovery Goals
Weight restoration	6:05 pm	Early–evening snack	2 servings of crackers, ¼ cup hummus	A	A	A	NA		None, yay!	Recovery goal met!
Weight maintenance	5:45 pm	Snack	Low-fat yogurt with fruit on the bottom	–	A	U	A ??		Restricted	Add granola to make this balanced. Ask RD if fruit on the bottom is a fruit serving
Metabolic balance	04:55	Late–afternoon snack	Apple, single-serve packet of mixed salted nuts	NA	A	A	A	40 minutes at gym		Yass!

Dinner

As the day winds down, our metabolism and brain waves do the same. The downward glide in energy distribution eventually makes sleep possible—and makes evenings challenging for people with eating disorders. For most bodies, optimal (but not required) dinner time is between 5:00 and 8:00. Eating after 8:00 isn't bad for you and won't keep your body from digesting dinner.

When a person's eating disorder plows through the body's "order of operations" guide rails, the crashes are severe. For instance, when a patient eats compulsively or restricts all afternoon, they are more likely to have confused hunger cues, cravings for foods, and inability to stop symptom use. Structure (when, what, and how much) is essential for nighttime eating.

One patient has a personal goal to lose weight and a busy work schedule. This gives him an almost daily excuse to skip mini-meal and an early-evening snack. He repeatedly tells me:

> Why do I have to eat in the afternoon if I'm not hungry? I have a handful of nuts around 4:00 or 5:00 sometimes, but I want to lose weight. So, I just can't justify eating when I don't want to.

I try my circadian rhythm talk. I preach about blood sugar. But it doesn't make a dent in the eating disorder thoughts or his chaotic afternoon meeting schedule.

By 6:00, he is exhausted, starving, and craving Indian takeout. His meal plan has weight maintenance ratios for his two favorite Indian dishes. but he's tired and annoyed, so he impulsively orders *both* matar paneer and chicken tikka masala, takes them home, and then eats way too much. He gets frustrated and purges. Then he heads to the gym to purge some shame from his psyche. When he gets back home, his shame and nutritional needs are still there. So, he binges on chips, salsa, and cookies right before bed.

We spoke many times about how blowing off afternoon eating events always set him up for chaotic eating disaster before, during, and after dinner. But the pattern continued.

One day, he had a 4:00 meeting outside of the office, where they offered an "appetizer" buffet. He gathered a few chunks of cheese, two handfuls of crackers, and a few pieces of dried fruit. He thought to himself: "I'll show Maria that eating in the afternoon won't make any difference in my evening." Then he sat down and ate during the meeting.

Back home, he prepared dinner and ate without too much of a hassle. He did not have his "regular" craving for ordering Indian food, so he didn't have to battle himself (and his eating disorder) over whether to order it.

Despite himself (or, in spite for me; I'm happy either way), he tried a new structured eating behavior at snack and dinner.

During our next session, he said: "You'll be proud of me. I ate a snack Wednesday and was able to eat my meal plan dinner that night without too much challenge." We went over his experience and I reiterated that metabolism science works regardless of whether or not your body can clearly communicate hunger signals.

Dinner Structure

Our culture tends to view dinner as the day's most "formal" and least rushed meal. It usually requires more preparation time. People tend to eat dinner with other people. Dinner norms often feel like impossible burdens and unreasonable expectations for someone with an eating disorder.

On the other hand, we remind our clients that dinner's characteristics mirror the traits of recovery-oriented meals:

- formal, as in, having *form*
- mindful preparation
- slower, calmer pace
- occasions to form and/or nurture human relationships.

Structured Eating de-escalates eating disorder thoughts and emotions by simplifying and demystifying dinner's form—starting with the plate itself.

We invite patients to imagine the empty plate as a blank canvas on which to visualize their next meal. We have three ways to "paint" the plate:

- plated meal: *separated* servings of each macronutrient. For example:

  - meatloaf, mashed potatoes, and string beans
  - salmon, yellow rice, and spinach
  - baked chicken, sweet potato, and broccoli.

- mixed meal: combining *all* macronutrients together. For example:

  - tomato sauce with meatballs and broccoli over spaghetti
  - shrimp and vegetable stir fry over rice
  - lettuce with steak, peas, green peppers, cheese, croutons, and salad dressing.

- contained meal: combines *some* macronutrients together, with the rest on the side. For example:

  - cheeseburger on a bun with a salad
  - chicken burrito with refried beans and guacamole on the side
  - grilled cheese sandwich and tomato soup.

Table 4.7 Meal Plan: Dinner

	Weight Restoration 3:2:1:2	Weight Maintenance 2:1:1:1	Metabolic Balance 1:2:1:2
Plated meal	6 oz grilled salmon with 2 Tbs creamy Dijon sauce, 1½ cups couscous, 2 cups green beans	3 oz grilled salmon, 2 Tbs creamy Dijon sauce, 1 cup couscous, 1 cup green beans	6 oz grilled salmon, 2 Tbs creamy Dijon sauce, ½ cups couscous, 2 cups green beans
Mixed meal	1 cup pasta noodles, 4 sausage links, 2 cups of salad with 2 Tbs dressing, and 1 bread roll with 2 tsp butter	1 cup pasta noodles, 2 sausage links, 1 cup of salad with 2 Tbs dressing	½ cup pasta noodles, 4 sausage links, 2 cups of salad with 2 Tbs dressing
Contained meal	Chicken quesadilla with ½ cup beans and ½ cup rice, ½ cup guacamole	Chicken quesadilla, ½ cup guacamole	Chicken quesadilla, ¼ cup guacamole

Dinner Meal Plans

We organized this sample dinner meal plan to show plated, mixed, and contained meals (Table 4.7).

When people in our care get the hang of Structured Eating, we must stay curious about their experiences and our blind spots. I'd watched my patient Leila make steady progress during six-plus years of sessions where we worked and ate together. A few months ago, when altering my appointment schedule, she and I discussed whether to continue our now twice-monthly sessions. She acknowledged her nutrition progress, but tried to explain why she needed to keep meeting:

> Maria, you are literally the only human I share meals with. I eat all my other meals alone. My anxiety and eating disorder talk me out of most, if not all, social experiences that involve food. I trust you, value the connection, and don't want to lose my only meal with someone else.

Her words surprised me. How had I not known this after six years? I had to stop and think hard about why I'd never picked up on—or asked about—this aspect of her life.

My life is filled with people: my children and husband, huge extended Italian families, friends, colleagues, and neighbors. I eat with people all the time. I don't regularly suffer from social anxiety, and when I am anxious, it doesn't affect my eating. Despite all I know about eating disorders, I struggled to wrap my mind around the fact that a patient never eats with anyone else but me. I hadn't fully realized how

Table 4.8 Food Log: Dinner

Goal	Time	Eating Experience	Food Consumed	C	P	F	F/V	Activity/ Exercise/ Movement	Symptoms	Recovery Goals
Weight restoration	7:30 pm	Dinner	2 Skinless chicken breasts, 4 cups of steamed vegetables	U	A	U	O	100 crunches	Over-exercise, restriction, filling up on vegetables	Less vegetables tomorrow for dinner, and add carbs
Weight maintenance	6:15 pm	Dinner	Burger with lettuce, tomato, and pickles, side salad with 2 Tbs dressing	A	A	A	A		None!	Completed dinner goal
Metabolic balance	8:00 pm	Supper	Chinese takeout: vegetable dumplings, container of beef lo mein	O	A	O	U	Walked home from friend's house	Emotional overeating	Talk to my RD about dinner strategies to avoid symptoms

completely her eating disorder and anxiety curtail her ability to make and keep connections.

Luckily, my new schedule had evening openings where we could focus on dinner. Straightaway, we began practicing "edgy" eating by giving her little challenges. The next time she visited her parents, she went out for dinner with them. When her next-door neighbor invited her to a potluck, she went.

As we ate mac and cheese together during our next session, she described an important connection with a colleague:

> You're going to be so proud. Gina asked me and another teacher to dinner and I said yes! It feels more important to connect with them than to give in to my anxiety *or* my eating disorder. But I'm still nervous because we're going to a Thai place and I'm not sure how to figure out portions.

At that session, we decided to have our dinner at a nearby restaurant to prepare for her new, exciting, and nerve-wracking social eating experience. From that session forward, we've ventured out together to practice eating in public and finding pleasure (and connection) while eating with friends, family and other people.

Dinner Food Logs (see Table 4.8)

Late-Evening Snack

The day's accumulated emotions, tensions, and anxieties can gush out in the evening. That means after dinner is prime symptom time for people with eating disorders. A *contained*, structured late-evening eating event is helpful, but often feels daunting.

Table 4.9 Meal Plan: Evening Snack

	Weight Restoration 2:2	*Weight Maintenance 2:1*	*Metabolic Balance 1:1*
Evening snack 1	2 cups cereal with 1 cup whole milk	1 cup cereal with 1 cup whole milk	1 cup cereal with ½ cup whole milk
Evening snack 2	1 banana, 3 Tbs chocolate-flavored nut butter, 1 cup juice	1 banana, 3 Tbs chocolate-flavored nut butter	1 banana 1½ Tbs chocolate-flavored nut butter
Evening snack 3	1 large bowl of tomato soup, 2 oz shredded cheese on top	1 mug of tomato soup, 2 oz shredded cheese on top	1 mug of tomato soup, 1 oz shredded cheese on top

Table 4.10 Food Log: Evening Snack

Goal	Time	Eating Experience	Food Consumed	C	P	F	F/V	Activity/Exercise/ Movement	Symptoms	Recovery Goals
Weight restoration	21:30	Nighttime snack	Oatmeal packet with a sprinkle of nuts	U	U	U	NA		Restricted portions	Add Boost before bed
Weight maintenance	22:10	Evening snack	Four bowls of raisin bran cereal with milk	O	O	?	O		Binge	Tomorrow play cards with Jim after snack
Metabolic balance	Midnight	Bedtime snack	Banana and 1 Tbs almond butter	-	A	A	A		Nope!	Nailed it! But need to work on sleeping

One strategy is to use balanced (and/or balanceable) snacks in *self-contained* packages. They already have their own structure.

For example, instead of having a large box of cereal in the house, have single-serving cereal cups. The patient adds milk to one cereal for a balanced pre-bedtime snack. A few other safe, balanceable self-contained foods: pudding cup, Chia Pod, yogurt cup, single-serving package of crackers with cheese or peanut butter, individual bag of Teddy Grahams, and so forth.

For patients on weight restoration plans, late-evening snacks may add necessary calories with supplements, like Ensure drinks and Boost.

Conclusion

Living all day with an eating disorder is brutal. It saps energy, disrupts metabolism, and activates the SNS. Its cunning, baffling, and powerful patterns feel like riding an endless rollercoaster. Grasping and using Structured Eating's details, timing, portions, and balancing can feel like an endless game of "whack a mole" for patients *and* clinicians,

Like other elements of treatment, Structured Eating can take months or years to master. But days aren't failures when clients use symptoms. If a client meets only the breakfast meal plan, we affirm how that breakfast will pave the way to more rewards today and tomorrow. While maintaining firm expectations, clinicians must also value and celebrate tiny, small, medium, and large successes.

We repeat: "Structured Eating gets a lot easier when you practice. Stick to the script and plan for more successful, balanced, and timely eating events."

People with eating disorders find it difficult to get through a day without resorting to symptom use. So, getting to a single bedtime symptom-free is an amazing accomplishment that nourishes a person's sense of hope.

Note

1 And when there is such a thing, my campaign team is ready!

5   Mindful Eating Foundations

When we shine the light of awareness on Structured Eating we catapult into the mysterious realm of mindfulness (or *misterioso mondo della consapevolezza*, as my Italian cousins would say).

Mindful Eating guides patients through an integrated progression of layering *awareness* onto Structured Eating. In some ways, this phase is "Structured Eating: Part Two." During Structured Eating's *mechanical* process, the body's ability to communicate and function increases. Mindful Eating moves our patients to *observation of the mechanical*—what we call mindfulness.

We guide clients to practice a level of presence that will simultaneously create containment and openness. Mindfulness embodies and contains experience, while opening clients to what is already present. Clinicians practice mindfulness too; honestly taking stock of our own expectations, stories, wishing to achieve the perfect session, and so on. When we witness (without acting *for* the client), we make room for their experience.

In yoga terms, practicing structure connects us with the material layer of our body. Mindfulness practice threads the vibrant layer of energy into our body. We awaken or reawaken sensations, notice our thoughts, become connected to our feelings, and notice other parts of the self that root us in profound presence.

We feel edges in the self—like how it feels when we stretch but can't quite touch our toes. As we practice exploring the edges, we expand our awareness and flexibility—stretching further to touch deeper parts of the self. Through mindful awareness of our body, we awaken *chi*, or life force— a life force essential to reaching our toes, recovery, and authentic living.

Flicking on the Light

Years ago, an Intensive Eating Disorder program invited me to introduce mindful meditation as a tool that clinicians could use to facilitate mindful eating. I was a well-seasoned eating disorder specialist, but a newly trained yoga therapist. I felt excited and worried about how fellow clinicians would receive this "yoga stuff." When the clinicians opened their eyes after the exercise, I saw a look of awe and wonder on many faces. They described a light going on inside them. They spoke of how readily they felt the embodied impact of the yoga practice. They were eager to know more about using grounding and mindful practices to help their own patients.

Scientific knowledge and yoga practice help patients transition to Mindful Eating. Depending on the meal plans and treatment goals, patients in Structured Eating practice "timing, timing, timing," or "balance, balance, balance" while they eat.

That's like learning to pat your head and rub your belly at the same time or juggling two balls in the air. It takes a lot of concentration at first—and gets easier with repetition. But there are still times when Structured Eating feels like juggling two balls in the air...in the dark. We know we're doing something, but we're not exactly sure what it is, or where we are.

When moving into Mindful Eating, patients don't lose, abandon, or scrap their "what and when" skills. Those skills provide essential data they use to learn the *additional* skill of noticing what they experience while doing their "whats and whens."

In Mindful Eating, people still juggle the two balls in the dark. But now, to observe how they do it, they turn on a flashlight *while* they juggle.

At first, they may hold the flashlight in one hand while juggling. This is awkward because it disrupts the juggling, leaving the balls (and probably the flashlight) on the floor. However, the practice is noticing what *does* happen and how they *experience* what happens (not "This doesn't work, so let's get rid of the flashlight. I'd rather keep juggling in the dark, so I don't have to see the balls on the floor").

When people with eating disorders first tiptoe into mindfulness, they often leap into hyper-vigilance, obsession, chaotic and perfectionist behaviors—or avoid the practice altogether. (That's also true for most people new to mindful practice, riding a bicycle, starting a new job, etc.) The tension, confusion, and uncertainty are natural, predictable, edgy, and organic for the journey of integrating new recovery skills.

So, clinicians need to be patient with clients while they practice. Trying to teach people in our care all the skills at once often leads to clinicians trying to juggle for them (and dropping more than balls and flashlights). That doesn't work very well—and defeats the purpose of mindful practice. It's their juggling, not ours.

Eventually, the juggling patient may try holding the back end of a small flashlight in their mouth, to free up both hands. This may improve the juggling, but their teeth and jaws aren't designed to grip a flashlight. Between the tension-generated pain and the instability of the "grip" (especially while juggling), the flashlight will drop on the floor. Even when that happens, clinicians coach clients to keep noticing what *does* happen and how we *experience* it, no matter what happens.

Over time, the patient juggler may discover other ways to shine light on their juggling act—for example, a headlamp. Whether attached to a coal miner's hard hat or a Nordic skier's cap, the headlamp frees up their hands and jaws—and considerable mental bandwidth. This provides a clearer view of the juggling act, and how the juggler *experiences* it. It also unlocks more of their life energy and uses it more efficiently.

Every time the client turns on a noticing light, they expand the breadth and depth of knowledge (or, if you will, data) about themselves, and access more life energy.

What People Don't Tell You about Mindfulness

What comes to mind when you hear the word "mindfulness"? A Tibetan monk sitting cross-legged in the Himalayan snow with a blissful countenance and a cup of tea? A long-haired New Ager in full lotus posture on a Tahitian beach chanting "oooohhhmmm" with a blissful countenance? (You get the idea.)

Well, in real life, practicing mindfulness isn't blissful. (Ignorance isn't bliss either, but that's another story.) Mindfulness takes work, and much more sustained practice than learning how to pronounce *consapevolezza* does.

Learning mindfulness is a challenge—even if your mind isn't already hijacked by an eating disorder.

Mindfulness is hard. It reminds me of writing this chapter on mindfulness. I am a certified yoga therapist, 200-hour Yoga Alliance registered yoga teacher and a Registered Dietitian with a Master of Science in both nutrition education and applied physiology from an Ivy League university. That didn't change the fear that I couldn't do this chapter right. I sat down at my desk to start several times. Instead of writing, I felt like crying.

Ironic? Not really—like mindfulness, writing *includes* fear and *requires* practice (and mindfulness).

Here's the irony. I finally started writing the chapter on an airplane, with two kids interrupting me every 30 seconds. (They were mine.) I felt frustrated, torn, and distracted.

I thought (but didn't vocalize) what I wanted to tell them: "Don't you know I'm a scientist, a yoga expert, and an eating disorders expert?! I need to do my work, and it's really hard, so stop acting like children who need their mother!"

A moment later, I felt chastened (while still frustrated) and thought to myself: "I can't write this chapter, much less this book. And if I do, will people think I know *anything* about mindfulness?"

As I noticed these distressing thoughts and emotions, I realized that I was practicing mindfulness.

Yes—even at 30,000 feet, sitting between two very antsy children—I noticed. Without lotus-posing (or leg room), I was aware. Being aware meant taking it all in: the plane, the kids, the chapter, my thoughts, and my feelings.

I then felt another important aspect of mindfulness: acceptance of what I'm noticing en route to a lovely destination while writing my book.

In other words, fellow passengers, the estimated time of departure—or arrival—for my mindfulness is right this second.

We all have unpleasant reactions to high-flying airplane inconveniences and down-on-earth mundane annoyances. They faintly mirror the reactions most of our patients have while moving into mindfulness.

Mindfulness is taking the next step of inhabiting one's body. "Inhabiting" goes beyond knowing that:

- We already live in our bodies.
- We need to be aware of what's happening around us (in case the pilot announces: "assume crash position!").
- We need to be aware of what's happening inside us (bladder alert; time to line up at the rear lavatory).

For people with eating disorders:

- "Becoming aware" can quickly signal "assume crash position!" reactions.
- "Becoming aware" usually involves waking up to pain and/or trauma.
- Mindfulness often means embodying agony and re-sensing anguish.

No wonder our patients resist *releasing* an eating disorder! For years, it's kept them "safe" by denying, distracting, detaching, and disassociating their body, thoughts, emotions, memories, trauma, and much more.

During the early steps of mindfulness, of course they'll want to run off and "assume crash position!"

There is profound irony and paradox here. People in the throes of eating issues are simultaneously detached from—and hyper-aware of—their body, food, and the experience of eating. Neither extreme facilitates mindful awareness.

As providers, we must remember what every person with eating disorders has at stake—and puts at risk—during treatment and recovery. When we engage in Mindful Eating we are asking our clients to:

- become more aware of how and what they are feeding their body
- become more aware of what *lies within* the body they are feeding.

In Structured Eating, patients may notice unwelcome noises in their body, such as hunger rumbles and gas. But in Mindful Eating, they begin to be present with their body's needs, demands, and urges. That's scary, uncomfortable, and unfamiliar territory to enter while still new to eating in a recovery-oriented fashion.

Asking our patients to become present to food, the experience of eating, and the experience of their body is like asking you or me to travel to a distant place where:

1. No one speaks or understands our language.
2. The currency isn't in multiples of 10; it's in multiples of *%@#y2K!?<.
3. The norms are unique to this culture (and indecipherable to us).
4. We feel so disoriented that we start to wonder if the air is green and the water is envelope. (Doesn't make sense? Welcome to wherever we are.)
5. And we've reached item number five before mentioning the food.

In short, the people in our care will often feel lost. We must notice and accept this reality. We reassure them (repeatedly) that feeling lost and afraid is natural, normal, and part of the journey.

Ask someone being chased by a tiger to notice their breath or consider their feelings. They'll run right by you, because they (literally) have something more important on their mind. The sympathetic nervous system keeps mindful awareness at bay. Mindfulness and active eating disorders symptoms cannot coexist in the same moment. Therefore, we have to practice one moment at a time.

Mindful Eating practice must go much deeper than gently raising a cup a tea to your mouth. It means leaning into our senses without trying to fix, change, or unplug from the experience. Mind and body must acknowledge each other's existence in relation to eating (and, ultimately, to everything else).

Mindfulness is the epitome of edgy for people in our care; people who must explore and expand their edges (or windows of tolerance) in order to heal.

Yoga helps patients notice the *body's* edges. Yoga also helps them use its language to invoke dialogue about *emotional* edges. You can't sink into the details of the experience when you've gone too far in a yoga stretch like the forward fold (otherwise known as trying to touch your toes). You're too busy managing your discomfort. On the other hand, a tiny stretch (like trying to touch your nose) won't provide enough sensation to capture your interest. Your body must engage in the stretch's edge before it can grab the subtle and valuable information mindfulness provides—and that you need to heal.

In yoga, our clients notice an edge through specific sensations like: "There's an intense pull in my left leg. It feels cool and warm at the same time. It's like lengthening and contracting at the same time. It feels challenging, but 'weirdly good.'" Practicing this language of physical noticing enhances our practice of experiencing and describing the edges of our emotional tolerance window.

We reiterate that mindfulness is necessary in recovery, it works, and it is worth practicing. We also remind them what people don't tell you about mindfulness: it is hard.

The Squatter at Home

Here's a thought experiment for you.

Imagine leaving your house for a couple of weeks. Your absence increases the odds that someone might break in and take some of your stuff. But your trip doesn't guarantee a burglary or turn someone into a burglar. If you leave for a couple of *years*, you don't guarantee that an uninvited squatter takes up residence in your home, or that some random person turns into a squatter. But your absence increases the "squatting" odds.

Now, imagine that a squatter does move into your home. Your only way to reclaim ownership is by busting through the door and demanding that the squatter leave. However, if you bust in alone, your odds of successfully (and safely) evicting the squatter and their debris plummet.

You'll need law enforcement, the courts, friends, a junk hauler, your insurance company, and/or other resources at your side. You're angry at the squatter for building a campfire on the rug and angry at yourself for not paying to keep the furnace on. With time and perspective, you may appreciate that the squatter (just barely) kept your house from burning down and kept some burglars at bay. But right now, in the moment of your return and your fury, you must acknowledge that:

- The unpleasant eviction process must start now, before the squatter *does* burn down your house.
- Trying to avoid the unpleasantries by cohabitating with the squatter doesn't work.
- Reclaiming your home will *not be painless or swift*.
- The process *will be worth the effort*.

An eating disorder is like a squatter taking up residence in the one place you live every day of your life: your body. The eating disorder misuses, abuses, and/ or demands ownership of your body, brain, thoughts, metabolism, relationships, spiritual wellbeing, capacity to feel, and more. When dislodging the disorder feels too overwhelming, "sharing" your space feels like the easier path.

But it doesn't work because an eating disorder doesn't share; its abuse of your body pushes you out to the curb. When "intolerable" feelings or situations arrive, an eating disorder screams: "Get out! This is my house now! I have squatter's rights." It incites you to abandon your authentic self through denial and/or dissociation from your feelings, your perception, and your body sensations. You may accede to its assertions and demands, thinking, "Maybe it's right. I don't belong here. It's too hard to live here now; I want to leave."

Meanwhile, the eating disorder squatter has no motivation to turn on the furnace and heat the whole house as long as its little indoor campfire stays lit. Denial, restricting, bingeing, purging, excess exercise, and so on are indoor campfires that simultaneously:

- just barely let you endure life difficulties
- endanger your body's survival.

The only way to reclaim ownership of your authentic self and your body from an eating disorder is to:

- Bust back into your body before it "burns down."
- Demand that the eating disorder leave.
- Begin taking up residence in your body.

It is virtually impossible to do any of this successfully or safely alone. You need the equivalent of law enforcers, junk haulers, and companions: therapists, dietitians, physicians, family, friends, spiritual advisors, colleagues, your insurance company, and/or other resources. You also need to know that, while the process will *not be painless or swift*, the process *will be worth the effort*.

Mechanical eating is like busting down the front door of your body. No matter what else is going on, you start to use the house again and prevent it from burning down. You begin to inhabit your body's spaces and find a safe room or two to use. This reduces room for the perpetrator, even though the perpetrator is still here.

You can't begin to recover your home unless you notice the burnt logs and other debris that the eating disorder left (or is still leaving) behind. Things are missing, broken, and misplaced. It's hard to look at all this mess. Very hard. It shows how much work you have to do.

You may not know where to start or recognize the safest rooms. You need (and *deserve*) other people's experience, guidance, patience, and support with the process. You need their faith that you can get through, and help you take things one room at a time; one piece of furniture at a time. You also need (and *deserve*) their willingness to hold you accountable when you want to give up and run away.

No matter what, moving in is essential if you want to reclaim the house— or your body—as your home.

In the Body

When clients arrive at our doors, they are sleepwalking (and perhaps having nightmares) in their bodies.

Back in Chapter 3, we described how active our body is, even when asleep: breathing, heart beating, blood circulating, nervous system signaling, brain operating, sleep cycles flowing, and so on.

Asleep, the body *also* interacts with the outside world. Don't believe it? List the times you remember waking up from a sound sleep in response to:

- hearing a fire alarm, siren, alarm clock, snoring (yours or someone else's)
- smelling odors from a skunk, something burning, flatulence (yours or someone else's)
- feeling an insect on your skin, nausea in your stomach, rain on your face
- seeing something in a dream or feeling something in a nightmare
- tasting the chocolate truffle your spouse gently placed in your mouth (OK; hasn't happened for me yet, but a girl can dream!).

With that in mind, I sometimes ask patients to:

- Think of the body as being "asleep" during Structured Eating—that is, operating in a mechanical, not-entirely-conscious way.
- Think of the body as "waking up" during Mindful Eating—that is, the underlying systems keep operating, while we notice them with steadily deepening consciousness.

Put another way: you may think that noticing changes nothing, and yet many things change. The way you engage with food, your body, and your symptoms change.

Crossing over from Structured Eating to Mindful Eating can take weeks, months, or years, depending on the person's capacity for presence and their ability to witness. We may not be able to identify the exact day or time the shift happens. But we notice language changing and experience changing. Eventually, the shift feels as palpable as waking up in the morning.

When do we lay on the layer of mindfulness? When the dietitian and the therapist think the patient is ready and brave enough to make the transition.

My colleague Rachel and I recently consulted about one of her patients, who is struggling with Mindful Eating. The patient said, "This is not a good time for me to do mindfulness work. I need to go back to Structured Eating, because I'm bingeing again."

During our discussion, Rachel and I explored the importance of helping patients interpret and frame Integrated Eating's phases or stages.

The Integrated Eating process isn't like driving down a hard and fast Interstate highway. Freeways have inflexible forks in the road with *large* directional signs you can see from a mile away. While in our care, people are not hopping between lanes on I-80 or exiting here (versus there) to take a sharp right turn on to Country Road 8904 in Iowa (or is it Idaho?).

Instead, during the Integrated Eating process, providers and patients explore where we are now (Interstate, country road, forest, swamp, quicksand, fog bank, up in the air, etc.). We practice active curiosity about what's missing and what's possible.

Rachel's patient still needs eating structure *and* she is ready to ask: "What is missing right now?" and "What is possible right now?" In her case, the answer (right now) is layering the awareness/witness consciousness on to Structured Eating. That's her path to practice and explore Mindful Eating.

That answer may look as simple as highlighting routes on a road map (remember paper road maps?). It isn't.

We repeatedly tell our patients that "this mindful stuff" calls them to stay connected with their bodies from the beginning to the end of eating event "trips" (and, eventually, other experiences). We reassure them that fear of traveling to unfamiliar territory (whether Iowa, Idaho, or India) is normal.

We acknowledge that symptom use may provide temporary relief from fear or discomfort. The eating disorder *seems* like a familiar, easy-to-use autopilot, even when part of us knows it drives us deeper into the swamp. We also acknowledge that they can't find recovery with the same old autopilot.

Let's be honest. Both clinicians and patients will feel tempted to search for shortcuts or get lost because recovery takes all of us over rough roads that seldom run in straight and predictable directions. Our hesitation is natural and understandable.

Rachel's therapeutic impasse reminded me of times I took shortcuts. I think of them as innocent collusions—*unnoticed* wishes my client and I shared:

- I don't want to be present to this messy and opaque process (so I avoid bringing up increased symptoms as a clinical issue).
- I do not want to sink into this moment's discomfort (so I avoid addressing resistance).
- I don't want to feel the pain of a broken body and spirit (so I tell myself: "It's not that bad" or "I've seen worse").

I colluded with denial and wishful thinking that my client (and I) would somehow "get it" without having to struggle with awareness. Wishing only to lean away from the mess, we played accomplices of the eating disorder and the stuck-ness.

Unfortunately, skipping, skimping on, or barreling through mindfulness (and the Mindful Eating phase) leaves people ill prepared (or, worse, unable) to travel the next part of their recovery journey. It dramatically increases their chances of getting lost ... and running back down the eating disorder highway to a hijacked home.

Yes, this process is tough. How do we as clinicians invite our clients and ourselves to walk this leg of the journey? By putting what we know into action. For instance:

- noticing and acknowledging (to ourselves and our patients) that this is hard
- accepting that this is hard
- accompanying them forward anyway—with invitation, guidance, attraction, support, and more
- embracing actions and attitudes which seem paradoxical, like patience and firmness
- holding hope for them in the moments when they can't do it themselves
- holding truth for them in the moments when they can't do it themselves
- staying in our bodies and practicing mindfulness.

Harder Than It Looks, Continued

During some morning in your past (whether 15 years or 15 minutes ago), you probably woke up late and rushed to get yourself ready to leave the house. You were flustered, scattered, and groggy. Next, you found yourself:

- in a crowded subway station, pushing through a crowd to cram into a train—hoping for at least enough room to breathe. Once you reach your stop, you run up the stairs and find yourself behind a pedestrian mob, waiting through two lights before you can cross a single intersection
- in a traffic jam, frantically trying to find a "fast" lane (that will get you to your exit approximately 2.5 seconds sooner than the car next door), breathing high doses of fumes and frustration. Once you reach your parking ramp, you run *down* the stairs and find yourself behind a pedestrian mob, waiting through two lights before you can cross a single intersection
- on a two-lane country road, stuck behind a school bus. You finally pass the bus, only to find yourself stuck behind a combine (top speed: 25 mph). You spend the rest of your ride growling to yourself: "Why isn't living in farm country *less* stressful?!"

Sound like something you've been through?

Now, imagine arriving at work or school to have me, your friendly yoga therapist, greet you at the door, and say:

- Notice your breath.
- Are you able to be with your physical sensations?
- Please get in touch with your deep-rooted feelings and your spiritual center.

Would that be ease-full for you? Or would you want to punch me in the nose?

When teaching meditation, I remind students how many things go on around and inside of us all the time. Even when sitting perfectly still, reading a book, we're "juggling" multiple balls:

- external stimuli: ambient noise, lighting, text on the page, how the page feels, etc.
- internal stimuli: thoughts, imagination, temperament, visualization, emotions, memories, breath, heart beat, etc.
- relationship stimuli: the reactions and responses between us, the internal stimuli, and the external stimuli.

Many everyday experiences take away stillness: work, traffic jams, arguments. In those moments, the stimuli we juggle seem more intense, complicated, frustrating, and difficult to discern.

In this agitated and frantic ball-juggling state, we will struggle to feel an obvious and accessible bodily sensation: breathing.

Good news: it is easy to learn how to notice our breath (plus, the benefits are almost immediate)

Less good news: it's hard to practice noticing in "real times" of traffic jams and such (but, the benefits are almost immediate!).

Bad news: we're unlikely to do the practice unless, for a moment, we intentionally stop juggling the balls (or turn on the headlamp while still juggling) and notice just one aspect of our experience (breathing).

Great news: you don't have to start breathing from scratch, or commute anywhere in search of an instructor. You and I have been breathing all along. We're breath masters. We were breathing before you started reading this book and before I started writing it. Can you notice if you're breathing now? Me too.

In mindfulness, the good news outweighs the bad news.

When we focus the bright light of "noticing" on one thing, our brain tends to "dim" the light we aim at other things happening at the same time. That's incredibly difficult to accomplish if your mind and body obsessively focus on your eating disorder.

But first, let's take a brain without an eating disorder. It is wired to:

- instantly stop hearing the car radio when we see another car about to hit us, and our sympathetic nervous system rushes our foot to the brake pedal

- stop feeling the breeze when we take our lover's hand on a walk
- instantly stop watching the TV when a dish crashes on the kitchen floor.

What happens when I notice less "dramatic" events, like breathing? I gather more information about my body and myself, and tend not to notice other things. Of course, the data about my rate and depth of my breath is there all along. But I cannot "read" the data unless I stop and shine a light of awareness on it.

The practice of mindfulness helps us connect with our senses, sensations, thoughts, feelings, breath, and emotions. The practice helps us identify our reactions when "stuck" behind a combine, in a traffic jam, and on the subway.

It works just as well in any situation. I have been known to exhale audibly during staff meetings. It reminds me how connecting to my breath helps me to acknowledge tension, anxiety, or impatience. It also helps me notice (and, ideally, soothe) my body's sensations.

Like staff meetings and eating events, mindfulness practice can be mundane and prosaic—and still generate insight. I'm reminded of a patient making a lot of progress in her recovery. She's mastered using her energy cues (tired, fatigued, mentally foggy, unable to focus, more anxious) as prompts to eat. In a recent session, she described a different sensation during her train ride home from work the night before.

> I was just sitting there and suddenly, I noticed a weird, foreign sensation in my stomach. It caught me completely off guard. I didn't recognize the sensation, so the experience was confusing and frightening.
>
> Then I said, "Oh, I think it's hunger." Right away, my next thought was, "Don't worry, it will pass." And it did.

This woman's hunger was there all along. Her new experience was an intersection of her body's material layer and her energy layer of awareness. Sitting still on the train, not being in her eating disordered thoughts, created space between the material and energy layers to collect the data.

This episode stands out because people with eating disorders rarely recognize basic and essential hunger and satiety cues. Even after finding reliable "time to eat" prompts, she was startled by a natural hunger signal from her body on that train. And even though she dismissed the sensation quickly and reactively, it opened a new chapter of necessary recovery work for us.

That story provided us both to dig deeper into key mindfulness questions, like "What is missing right now?" and "What is possible right now?"

The recovery process repeatedly calls people to dig deeper. Throughout treatment, we're asking each patient to do things the hard way, because that is the path of healing. The healing hard way includes painful, slow, and "worth-it" practices of connecting/reconnecting with their body, mind, soul, and authentic self.

What Do I Notice and How Do I Know?

When we shine the light of awareness on to eating events, our patients begin noticing how compromised their bodies are. For instance, ongoing restriction can blunt *hunger* signals while overeating and bingeing may blunt *fullness* cues. Mindfulness creates openings to help our patients practice ways to tolerate what they find and move toward acceptance of what the eating disorder has done and is doing now.

Mindful Eating is hard work for people with eating disorders, because they all have different ways of understanding awareness. Therefore, clinicians must be sensitive to, and start teaching from, where the patient's understanding is now—even if they are disconnected from their embodied experiences and sensations.

Indeed, they need lots of practice to notice their five senses.

The first questions we explore in mindful eating are:

- What do I notice about the food I'm eating?
- How do I know what I'm noticing?

Our senses help us answer these questions for ourselves with food every day, if we notice.

In yoga therapy, I ask my patients, "What do you notice and how do you notice it?" If they tell me, "I feel a pain in my back," I dig deeper with a scientific inquiry: "Tell me more about *how you know* it's pain; describe the sensation of pain in this moment." In other words, what data provides you with the evidence that it's pain?

This approach leads clients away from being swallowed up by the pain (or other difficult sensation) by leading them toward curiosity and inquiry.

We use the same tactics in a meal support. When someone says they feel hungry or full, we invite more information: "What sensations do you have right now? How about thoughts or feelings? Tell me more about how you know this."

This kind of mindful dialogue invites patients to:

- gather data about their experience through mindful noticing
- accurately identify their experience by using awareness-illuminated evidence
- lean deeper into their experience, and accurately identify additional evidence revealed during deeper exploration.

The holistic process of exploring the origin of one's observation illustrates what science tells us about mindfulness' influence on neurobiology.

When we repeat a pattern of behavior, thinking, or feeling (such as eating disorder symptomatology), our neuroplastic brains create and/or deepen neural pathways like a monster truck leaves tracks in the mud. Staying in our muddy metaphor, mindfulness lightens the tire tracks by morphing the monster truck into a car. Further practice can morph the car into a child's wagon which leaves barely a trace.

Perhaps, with continued practice, a green pasture will grow in this muddy acre while we're busy making tracks in new fields. You may remember that the pasture once was mud, but now the pasture feels peaceful.

Mindfulness practice stimulates neuroplasticity to simultaneously:

- create and/or deepen new and/or healthier neural pathways
- reduce the tendency to revisit (and reinforce) the existing, problematic neural pathways.

Exploring with Senses

The five senses bring awareness to any life event. When we proactively put them to work before, during, and after eating events, they become our mindful data collectors. With the senses, Mindful Eating techniques and practices help patients get more intimate with the food and their bodies.

During the Mindful Eating phase, we guide people through meals and snacks with multiple prompts. Table 5.1 includes common prompts, and actual patient responses.

The noticing practice in Table 5.1 is quite basic. However, even basic noticing *momentarily* interrupts the eating disorder's imperative of instant avoidance/relief/gratification, and so on, and challenges eating disorder patterns. Those mindful moments help unstick problematic neural pathways and cultivate new ones.

The specificity of this approach guides patients to focus on *one* thing already happening in their eating moment. Our experience shows that people with eating disorders learn to eat mindfully by:

- using senses to bring attention to a specific quality of the food
- holding that attention for a sustainable moment
- noticing how the body, emotions, thoughts, and beliefs respond to the sensation.

For instance, I recently brought raw baby carrots, pear, avocado, and snap peas to my appointment with an anxious patient with avoidant restrictive food intake disorder (ARFID). We did a food exposure sense check with each item.

Table 5.1 Provider Prompts

Provider Prompts	Patient Responses
Notice your breath (a basic yoga practice)	Very shallow and very tense
Can you see the food? Can you look at it closely?	• I see the food. It looks like too much • I see the food. It's not enough • I see the food. It looks gross But I know I feel like that before every meal. I remember that my RD [Registered Dietitian] says I'm feeding my body the amounts it needs
What qualities of the food do you see?	I see fluffy eggs, dry toast. and wet, fresh fruit
Can you bring it up to your nose? What does it smell like? Does it remind you of anything?	I smell the essence of the grapefruit first. Then the smell of toasted bread. My mom used to make me toast with butter before school when I was young. I used to love that breakfast and now I hate it
Can you put it in the palm of your hand or hold it with your fingers? What's the texture like? Does it remind you of anything?	The dry toast is rough. It needs butter but I'm afraid to put it on. The eggs are slippery; that's gross. The grapefruit is juicy; too messy. The grapefruit pieces remind me of rain drops
What specific sounds does the food make as you're eating it? How did that sound the same or different from other foods you're eating at this meal?	The toast crunches and is louder than the eggs. I almost feel like I can hear the grapefruit bursting in my mouth when I chew it
What do you notice about the textures and taste this food provides?	I feel the crunchy texture of the toast. It's kind of chewy and crunchy at the same time. The butter tastes good, but it scares me because it'll make [or keep] me fat. The eggs don't really have a taste in comparison to everything else. They kind of blend in. The grapefruit is juicy and exploding with taste in my mouth

She had no problem with the appearance, texture, smell, and taste of every food but the carrot. She had no problem with the carrot's appearance, texture, or smell. But when she bit into it, her experience changed. She said, "The taste is OK, but chewing it reminds me of chewing rubber. That felt gross, so I had to spit it out."

This data prompted us to include all these foods except the carrots in her week's meal plan. We agreed to repeat the carrot sense test the following week. We tried vegetable fried rice with cooked carrots. Unfortunately, she refused the carrots in this form, too.

It bears repeating: This is *not* an easy process.

6   Mindful Eating in Real Life

As you may recall from ninth-grade chemistry, the scientific method is a two-phase process. The second phase builds upon the first.

1. It begins with systematic observation, measurement, and experiment.
2. It continues with the formulation, testing, and modification of hypotheses.

We invite patients to practice systematic observation and measurement of their experience during Mindful Eating. We frame mindfulness questions as exercises in simple curiosity. This can help defuse some of the fear, anxiety, and other resistance.

Patients begin replicable experimentation (informed by systematic observation and measurement) as they transition into the next phase. During Intuitive Eating, they continue experimenting—and practice how to formulate hypotheses about the data they discover, test the hypotheses, and then modify them.

Mindful practice is simply noticing—not assigning judgment, interpretation, or other value to what we notice. To paraphrase a wonderful psychology truism: we're guiding patients to be more curious than furious.

And, to paraphrase a yoga truism: no teacher can teach you to move mindfully in your body the way your body will teach you how to move mindfully.

The Structure of Mindful Eating

Wait, didn't we leave structure behind a couple of chapters ago? Not entirely.

Remember that Mindful Eating layers awareness on to what clients learn during Structured Eating. Hence, we continue using meal plans as essential tools. (Some people need, move into, and practice Mindful Eating, even though they are on the tail end of a nutritional goal.)

We ask patients to visualize the transition from Structured to Mindful Eating like a cable channel guide. The guide provides utilitarian data about dozens (or hundreds) of choices. But it isn't a TV show. Is the guide data useful to you? That depends on whether you:

1. scroll with your remote, "open" a channel, and *watch* a real TV show
2. push the off button on your remote.

Structured Eating's eating events are also utilitarian. They aren't full recovery, but they contain data (and food). Unlike a channel guide, the food is useful to your body no matter what else you do. The data? That's only useful if you "select the channel" and *watch* your eating events.

Fortunately, we can't misplace our body between the couch cushions the way we can with the remote. Our body is always with us—including eyes, nose, ears, tongue, and nerve endings that let us sense what's happening when we eat.

In Mindful Eating, we invite patients to:

• bring their senses to the table and observe multiple aspects of the eating experience
• explore how feeding the body relates to body sensations and behavior (like hunger and fullness cues, flatulence, etc.).

We start with concrete *and* open-ended questions. One patient calls the questions "simple, but deceptively complex."

1. What do you notice about the timing or pacing of your eating events?
2. What is the energy around your eating events? Are you rushing, on the go, frantic, calm, detached, foggy, distracted?
3. Who do you eat with?
4. How many of your eating events are prepared at home, eaten out, takeout, etc.?
5. How do you connect with food? What do you know about you and your relationship to food? What do you like? What do you dislike? Do you use your senses at the table?
6. What is your relationship to hunger and fullness?
7. Other.

Mindful Eating provides a wider perspective by layering on questions of noticing and clarification. Our dialogue deepens when we ask our patients to consider:

• *How I eat* (pacing, timing, energy, manipulating food, ability to stay present, conversing with other people present, not conversing with other people present, etc.)
• *Where I eat* (in my room, at work, standing in the kitchen, at a restaurant, at the TV/computer, while driving, etc.)

- *Who I eat with* (no one, other people, with the eating disorder, etc.)
- *How I acquire food* (noticing my relationship to shopping, finding, buying, ordering in, taking out, etc.)
- *How I prepare and present food I eat* (preparing, cleaning, cooking, arranging dishes and glasses on the table, etc.)
- *How my body responds during this eating event* (over-full or under-empty sensations, distraction, anger, calm, flatulence, purge urges, fear, growling stomach, fed, nausea, anxiety, satisfaction, distended stomach, energized, resentment, etc.)
- *How my body responds after this eating event* (over-full or under-empty sensations, distraction, anger, calm, flatulence, purge urges, fear, growling stomach, fed, nausea, anxiety, satisfaction, distended stomach, energized, resentment, etc.)

Fullness and Hunger

It's hard to make sense of new (or old) data unless we organize the information in ways we can understand. For example, most eating disorder treatment programs use some variation of a hunger and fullness scale.

I ask patients to use hunger and fullness scales in the same way they use a stereo's volume control (10 tiny lines painted the edge of a knob or 10 tiny lights on a digital display). In addition to raising and lowering the decibels coming through the speakers, those little lines provide a visual representation of the stereo's:

- current sound level
- potential sound level (up or down).

Mindful Eating clients use hunger/fullness scales in their food logs and journaling practice—to help them mindfully discern what they are sensing when they are super-full, super-hungry, and/or somewhere in between. The scales help them (and us) to:

- monitor (and notice) the current moment
- monitor (and notice) change from past moments
- consider potential changes in future moments.

Our rating scale uses these 11 "volume" lines:

1. starving
2. intense hunger
3. very hungry
4. hungry
5. slightly hungry
6. neutral

7. slightly full
8. full
9. very full
10. intense fullness
11. stuffed.

We make regular use of Chapter 5's "prompts" chart (Table 5.1).

Food Logs

Because eating disorders foster obsession, people in our care need skills, guidance, and practice to identify the difference between awareness and super-hyper-rigid focus. As clinicians, we must keep our eyes out for moments and methods the eating disorder uses to trick our clients into believing they are being mindful when, in reality, they are distorting or obsessing.

During Structured Eating, food logs give patients a structure to track the timing, balance, and amounts of eating events. It makes room for sensation, but that's not the primary focus.

During Mindful Eating, we expand food logs to help patients remember (and re-notice) the new data gathered through their senses. The log's directive, guiding structure provides daily practice in *observing* body sensations, emotions, and thoughts. The logs help reveal a holistic picture of their recovery-focused experience *and* their eating disorder-focused experience.

The food log in Table 6.1 tracks a whole day for a client with restrictive bulimia. Their goal is weight maintenance. During Mindful Eating, they are still battling compulsive exercise and urges to purge.

When reviewing a log like this with a client, the dietitian would:

- remind them of the "eat within first hour" rule
- help them plan a pre-workout snack
- remind them that lunch was balanced
- set (or reinforce) exercise parameters/limits
- discuss pacing during and between eating events
- go over their next meal plan.

One of my patients stuck to a rigid meal plan for fear that he would binge. His food log showed that he weighed cheese portions to keep them under two ounces. When I asked him about it, he said weighing cheese kept him from bingeing, and then having to purge.

I challenged him to observe whether he was responding to physical cues or to a mental construct. He admitted that it *might* be a mental construct. I suggested that the mental construct *might* be constructed by his eating disorder.

Table 6.1 Food Log: Weight Maintenance, All Day

Event Time	Event	Pre-eating Event Intention	Food Consumed	C	P	F	F/V	Hunger/ Fullness (Before/ After)	Pacing: Fast (F) Moderate (M) Slow (S)	Symptoms	What I Noticed	What's Next Intention	Action Plan
5:45 am	Wake									Restict	I noticed I was hungry in class	Feed myself!	Eat snack as soon as I leave here!
06:30	Spin class	Enjoy class									Judgemental thoughts comparing my body to others in the class	Practice riding within my edge, body acceptance	Next week take more breaks in spin class when tired
07:30	Snack	Honor hunger	Apple	NA	U	U	A	0/3	F	Unbalanced snack	I was rushing and very hungry and inhaled the apple	Eat breakfast as soon as I get to work	Plan and pack a balanced snack before class
08:00	Breakfast	Feed body well after exercise	Bowl of Special K cereal, 2% milk, big handful sliced almonds, orange juice	A	A	A	A	1/6	F	NA	Noticed the sweetness of the OJ, felt energized after eating	Practice acceptance: I was still hungry	Eat snack by 11am

Time	Type	Plan	Food					Date		Behavior	Notes	Skill	Outcome
10:50 am	Snack	Slow down pacing		A	A		NA	2/6	M	No	Ate more slowly, feeling anxious about how much I need to get done today	Put my body's needs first	Eat lunch in afternoon meeting
13:30	Lunch	Go with the flow—eat what they are serving at meeting	2 slices of pizza, salad with dressing	A	A	A		2/8	F	Urge to Purge	Feel very full and uncomfortable about what I ate	Ride the wave of urge	Stay in meeting, text my friend and let her know I'm having a difficult time. DO NOT GO TO BATHROOM!
05:00	Mini-meal	Follow my meal plan	Yogurt, granola bar, banana	A	A	U	A	3/7	S	Avoiding eating	Still had thoughts about how much I ate at lunch. Noticed banana was a bit mushy	Bring ease into ED thoughts	Did some breathing
8:00 pm	Dinner	Eat all components	Steak salad with dressing, one piece of bread (did not eat bread, ate half salad)	U	U	U	A	2/7	M	Restrict	Thoughts were intense. I noticed how much resistance I had to eating all my dinner.	Trust that the food is not too much	Add extra carb, protein and fat to my evening snack to make up for restrictive portions

(Continued)

Table 6.1 (Cont.)

Event Time	Event	Pre-eating Event Intention	Food Consumed	C	P	F	F/V	Hunger/Fullness (Before/After)	Pacing: Fast (F) Moderate (M) Slow (S)	Symptoms	What I Noticed	What's Next Intention	Action Plan
10:30	Evening Snack	Eat mindfully	1 slice of bread (added carb), 3 Tbs of peanut butter (added one more to make up for dinner), and an apple	A	A	A		3/7	M	No!	Noticed the texture of crunchy apple with creamy PB	Get to bed	Start evening bedtime routine
11:00 pm	100 crunches									Compulsive exercise	I was checked out and found myself doing crunches wildly	Stop doing crunches	Plan a rest day tomorrow

We returned to my message that recovery is about living in his body, not in his mind. It took several years for this truth to penetrate, so I needed patience and persistence. I also needed the food log data.

For example, when a person logs "There was a ton of oil on my vegetables," we ask them to snap a few photos of the vegetables, so we can discuss it together. Usually, we discover that the eating disorder distorted the amount of oil (or other food). When we notice together and individually, the client strengthens their recognition muscles. Also, when they note eating disorder phenomena like "portion distortion," we notice (and acknowledge) their noticing progress.

We can't expect that noting the behavior will change it, but we can remind patients that they are practicing how to get a better grip on reality-based thinking.

We do expect that the eating disorder will repeatedly try to hijack food logs (and often succeed) in order to reinforce symptoms. Despite this, food logs are still radically helpful.

We also must expect that people will resist using the logs because:

- They are sick of it.
- It takes a lot of time.
- They don't want to be mindful.
- It doesn't feel like it's helping enough or soon enough.
- It feels like it's reinforcing their food rigidity.
- "It keeps me in my head, not my body." (In other words, the eating disorder is distorting the tool.)
- The eating disorder is working to keep them stuck.

For the dietitian, all of these reactions are information we can and must use. We can discuss and use all of it to support our patients' recovery. We can use our curiosity, asking questions like: "What's making you sick of it?"

We can also help them ride the wave by, for a day or two:

- filling out fewer columns
- logging every other day
- logging fewer eating events
- taking a break from all logging
- checking in with us at the end of the day, instead of logging
- snapping and sending a photo of the food, instead of filling out the food columns.

We nutritionists must be on our best game each and every time we view the logs—and every time we don't get a log. We must be willing to have the next conversation, no matter what.

For instance, when we don't have the log, we do a mindful "food recall" for the past 24 hours or the entire week. We ask them to notice the experience of not being able to recall the experience of eating a vegetable 144 hours ago. Then, we reinforce that we can't practice mindfulness without using noticing tools—and the food log is our primary, most effective tool.

Noticing Before, During, and After

Mindful Eating must include the moments before, during, and after each eating event. In those moments, we give patients two goals:

1. Observe your state: your inner and outer environments.
2. Eat anyway.

Below are simple questions and statements we deploy to prompt patients' mindful noticing and observation. Whatever our patients notice, we respond by calmly validating and encouraging their noticing by saying, "yes, this is your body communicating with you."

Of course, just because clients notice something doesn't mean they're ready to respond to it.

Let's mindfully think back to waking up in the morning. Shifting from its sleeping/fasting state, the body desperately needs nutrients to replenish and to engage its systems to work properly. Brain waves speed up. These many morning transitions may wreak havoc on a patient's physical and emotional body—leaving people more susceptible to anxiety, panic, depression, or trauma responses.

We encourage them to eat anyway because feeding their body in the morning is not optional. The mindful eater can notice their body's cues (e.g., hunger cues) and their emotional state (e.g., anxiety) *and* eat a balanced meal.

Did we mention? This is *not* an easy process!

Before

*   Think of the fullness/hunger scale. Where do you sense that *your body is* right now on the scale?
*   What else are you noticing about your body right now? (e.g., starving, nauseous, tense, etc.)
*   Take a moment to notice your feelings right now. Some may be easy to access because they're right on the surface, while others may be more hidden or tucked away.

During

- Notice your breath (a basic yoga practice).
- Can you see the food? Can you look at it closely?
- What qualities of the food do you see?
- Can you bring it up to your nose? What does it smell like? Does it remind you of anything?
- Notice your pacing. What data is it providing?
- Notice what you are and aren't doing with the food while it's on your plate. What data does that provide?
- Notice what you are and aren't doing with the food while it's in your mouth. What data does that provide?

After

- Notice your breath. What's it like now?
- What kinds of sensations are you having in your body?
- Notice any thoughts. Let's give them the microphone for a moment. They want to be noticed. In this moment, your *only* job is to simply observe them, not do anything else.
- What are you feeling? Do you notice any emotions?
- Where in your body do you notice this feeling?
- Notice fullness level. What can you tell me about how you experience your fullness?
- How are your senses informing you about your experience?

Again, our job is to calmly validate and encourage their noticing. We hold the space for the impact of their experience, without trying to fix it or change it. We must also make space for the intensity *we* feel. This demands that we embody and attune to our own experience.

- When a patient says I feel _____, we ask: "To what extent can you stay with this feeling so you can gather its data or information?"
- When someone says I feel _____, we ask: "Where do you feel that right now in your body? Where is it inhabiting space in your body?"
- When someone is feeling intensely, we ask: "Are you within your edge or over the edge?"

The noticing is basic *and* it presents a major challenge to the eating disorder's self-harming pattern and imperative of instant avoidance/relief/gratification, and so on.

The post-meal check-in (aka, noticing) is a fertile moment for patients to put their data to use. We ask them to let "what I just noticed" inform an action plan for the next period of their day, and, if possible, inform their next eating event. In other words, "what happens next after what just happened."

What happens when a Mindful Eating day goes off the rails? Informed by training and experience, clinicians acknowledge that the most valiant efforts to eat in a connected and mindful way may not turn out the way we hoped. Nevertheless, they always have data.

Perfectionism-prone people with eating disorders often can't tolerate mishaps and mistakes, and react by denigrating or denying "mistake data." We remind patients that data is "bad" only when it's inaccurate.

"Mistake data" is fuel for many transformative moments. Just visualize a toddler learning to walk. In the beginning, they fall down and resort to crawling (standing mistakes!) before they can stand up on their own. They fall down and resort to crawling (walking mistakes!) much more often than they toddle. They shuffle and fall down (walking mistakes!) before they can walk steadily. They walk fast and lose their balance (running mistakes!) before they can run.

Without making hundreds of mistakes, the toddler can never learn to walk or run, because:

- The child can't adjust to the "mistakes" if they don't notice/experience them.
- Their brain cannot create the balance and movement neural pathways it needs to engage the body in the practice of walking.
- Their body cannot create the muscle memory and coordination it needs to engage in the practice of walking.
- The child can't access the instinctive body wisdom wired into every living thing.

We remind them that "mistake data" is fuel for many transformative moments. Then, we repeat.

Into Action

After practicing Structured Eating for many months, one of our patients started to notice familiar sensations (urge to purge) and a new sensation (eagerness to move past the eating disorder). While discussing her food log entries, Michele, her dietitian, suggested additions to where and what to eat. When they reached dinner planning, however, the patient stubbornly resisted every suggestion. She said: "By the end of the day, I feel I've done all I can handle for one day and I … well … I'm done."

In effect, she was saying, "By dinner time, I'm over my edge." Michele responded by metaphorically giving the client "permission" to step back from the edge, for now.

REGISTERED DIETITIAN (RD): Here's my observation, or theory. Right now, you're noticing a meaningful edge in your daily recovery. Does that come close to describing what you're experiencing?

HER: Well, I think that nails it.

RD: OK. So, for the next few days, let's practice noticing that edge every evening—and see what data you can gather about that edge.

HER: Hmm. Frankly, I'd much rather avoid feeling it or thinking about it.

RD: I hear you. Remember, that's why we call it an edge; it's edgy.

HER: I suppose.

RD: I suppose so, too. *For now*, we won't ask you to change what you're doing in the evening. Let's add to lunch and snacks to help your body get what it needs, while you gather your edge data.

HER: OK.

RD: Let's both think of the data as something we'll use to inform what we do next week after 4:00 pm. I can hear that this is something you can do until our next session.

HER: OK. I will. Thank you for understanding.

RD: Hey, that's what noticing and mindfulness lead to: understanding!

Michele practiced containing and giving space to the experience of recovery and eating, while still communicating firm expectations for recovery eating. Witnessing our patient's edges helps us be mindful of intense feelings that might otherwise be misinterpreted as resistance.

Clinicians must address the stubborn, edgy, and devious resistance known as denial. We often gather data about client denial when the logs say one thing, but their body tells us something quite different. These moments help us to address denial with data about reality.

My patient Sarah's metabolic balance food logs consistently showed her following her meal plan. She wondered why she wasn't yet seeing some weight loss. Instead, she gained some weight, felt frustrated, and began questioning the treatment.

While suggesting the possibility that her set point had changed, I also sensed that her reporting wasn't completely accurate. Not because she was trying to hide anything from me, but because she wasn't ready to face eating for herself.

I consulted with Sarah's therapist, who began a long stretch of deeper emotional work with Sarah. That work informed our nutrition work. As Sarah faced scarier parts of herself and addressed her shame, denial diminished in our conversations. She began honestly admitting: "I am always thinking about food" and "If I have to give up eating certain things then I'd rather stay this size." I validated how wonderful her honesty was, and how hard it is to honestly express what's really happening.

One of our weight restoration patients kept meticulous food logs showing little or no exercise on days filled with meals, mini-meals, and snacks. Yet, she was losing weight. When the nutritionist asked, the patient denied exercising. The nutritionist questioned portions and the patient repeatedly said she was eating everything on her plan. The nutritionist then calmly and directly addressed what she saw.

> Look, this just doesn't add up. Actions speak louder than words. You're losing weight. I see evidence that something is getting overlooked. As your body's advocate, you and I need to talk about whatever it is. You're telling me you're eating the same and not exercising. I have to ask you again if we are missing anything.

The patient continued to deny hiding or omitting information.

For several more weeks, the nutritionist spoke directly about the patterns she observed. Finally, the patient admitted that she was obsessively exercising and restricting. She said: "I'm running every morning. When I tell you I ate a sandwich, I don't tell you it's on light bread with the crusts cut off." Clinicians must be persistent, patient, and trust what we observe.

Our patients are deeply habituated to let eating disorder thoughts run the show before, during, and after eating events. So, we intentionally invite their eating disorder thoughts out into the light. We commonly hear things like:

• Well, I'm afraid that I'm not going to get through this meal.
• I can't even imagine how I can keep from purging when I'm done eating.
• I'm scared of this food.
• This is not enough food. It will never be enough, and I'll be miserable for hours afterward.

We don't ask (or expect) patients to *act on* these thoughts. We ask that they notice.

The Mindful Eating phase also makes room for the feelings swirling around eating events. This part of the process opens the door to noticing additional things.

ME: How do you feel right now?
THEM: I feel really anxious.
ME: OK, how do you know that you are feeling anxious?
THEM: I feel like I can't really get a breath in. And, at night, I feel my heart rate race.
ME: That's good; you noticed concrete and recognizable data provided by your body.
THEM: I guess so, but what good is that? You haven't fixed me or told me what to do instead. I still feel anxious!
ME: I know. The data is additional information that you didn't notice before or noticed sporadically. We can't change what's happening in there

until we know what's happening in there. To know, we have to collect the data without judging it or freaking out about it. For now, it's enough that you *only* notice it.

When Yoga Walks into a Meal

Because people with eating disorders usually feel disconnected from their bodies, clients practice gathering more data about their body—especially during meals, mini-meals, and snacks. We guide the practice with statements like these:

- Rub your hands together for 10 seconds, and then put them on your lap.
- Rub your hands together for 10 seconds, and then touch your chair.
- Take off your shoes and place your feet flat on the floor. Then, close your eyes and feel the ground or floor for 15 seconds.

Clinicians can deepen this centering/noticing practice in meal support groups or treatment center eating events. Once the patients are grounded, we do a simple breathing exercise to bring awareness to the body—and containment to the person. Next, we move into about five minutes of noticing sensations, thoughts, and emotions.

We close this short group or individual meditation by asking participants to create an intention. This simple combination of actions usually creates a palpable sense of presence in the room—before anyone begins to eat.

People with trauma history and dissociative episodes are drawn to the safe containment that this pre-meal practice can provide. Some of our patients use it regularly during other meals when they feel close to dissociation.

In the Structured Eating chapter, I mentioned a patient convinced that leaving her apartment clean before work is more important than eating breakfast. During sessions with our program's meal support coaches, we observed that she was very anxious, wanted to get through the meal quickly, and therefore ate rapidly.

When I shared this observation, she said: "Yeah, I want this to be over. Like, I can't connect to my body right now. I do not want to be here doing this. I guess that's why I'm rushing."

However, the patient ate incredibly slowly when sharing breakfast with her therapist! The therapist and I agreed that swift and slow eating both reinforce the patient's body disconnection.

She disconnected from her body for fear that intense feelings would prohibit her from getting through the meal. Understanding this apparent fast–slow contradiction helped everyone on the treatment team to train the patient in awareness and presence while eating. This helps her develop moderately paced eating—which creates space to notice and connect with her body.

One common yoga therapy scenario provides a good example of facilitating mutual data access. During a stretch, a client may say: "I'm feeling sad." I will ask: "Where in your body are you feeling that sadness?"

THEM: It's deep in my chest.

ME: Can you stay with the feeling of sadness in your chest and describe the sensation of "sad"?

THEM: No, it's too much. I just can't.

ME: OK, it sounds like you're over your edge. (*I'm aiming to help the person walk away from the edge, while continuing to gather data.*)

THEM: Yes. Yes, I am.

ME: OK, what's happening with your breath? Tell me with words what you notice about your breath. (*I'm aiming to help the person walk away from dissociation and stay in their body to gather data about things other than being at the edge.*)

THEM: It's hard.

ME: I know. Let's take a breath. Now, can you notice your breath, your physical sensations, thoughts?

THEM: My breath is shallow. My chest feels tense and my thoughts are racing.

ME: OK, breath shallow, chest tense, thoughts racing.

THEM: Yes.

ME: Say more about what you notice about the sad?

THEM: I can see it as dark gray and heavy; it's almost throbbing.

ME: Good. Can you connect the information to something happening in your life now?

THEM: I think so, a little bit. I feel this kind of sad when my mother doesn't call every day. It's like she abandons me.

ME: It sounds like this sadness is connected to abandonment.

THEM: It certainly does.

Her ability to witness her edge and observe the "sad" naturally begins the *process of processing* the emotion and experience. Rather than invite indescribable feelings that overwhelm a person, we invite them to observe the edge (e.g., deep in my chest) with a minuscule change in perspective (while noticing my breath). We didn't jump over the edge and plummet down. We tiptoed up to the edge, stepped back, and noticed. This safe, contained yoga practice produced valuable data.

Mindfulness practice gives our clients a safe way to ride the waves of the sympathetic nervous system while staying in their body. As in the "sad" example above, mindfulness practices like yoga provide non-verbal ways to acknowledge our experience. Mindfulness helps people resist bingeing, restricting, purging, compulsive exercise, and more.

However, we *don't* deny, dismiss, or take them out of their experience. We understand that they *are* safe when they have "big scary" feelings. Mindfulness practice doesn't buy into the eating disorder's melodrama. Mindfulness undermines the belief that feelings are dangerous or bad. Instead, it helps clients embody the truth: feeling is.

Practicing mindful observation steadily increases the person's level of tolerance for discomfort. A sustained practice of noticing expands (often incrementally) their capacity to expose themselves to uncomfortable feelings—and their ability to explore them with curiosity.

Mornings

As we discussed in earlier chapters, morning anxiety is common for people with eating disorders. Integrated Eating's roots in science and yoga give us several options when responding to resistance, including mindful body practices and food strategies.

I work with a boy in his teens with avoidant restrictive food intake disorder (ARFID). His morning anxiety creates a decrease in appetite, blunted hunger cue, and early fullness. As a result, he has difficulty eating the full amount of his morning food.

I taught him a *pranayama* (breath practice) to use:

- before he sits down to eat
- when he feels anxiety while eating
- when he resists finishing a meal due to anxiety.

Table 6.2 Meal Plan, Morning

	Weight Maintenance 2:1:1:1	*Metabolic Balance 1:2:1:2*
Breakfast 1	1 cup of dry oatmeal cooked with 1 cup 2% milk, 2 Tbs nuts, ½ box raisins	½ cup of dry oatmeal cooked with 1 cup 2% milk, 2 Tbs nuts, 1 box of raisins, 1 hard-boiled egg
Breakfast 2	2 large pancakes, 2 sausage links, 2 tsp butter, 2 Tbs syrup, ½ cup strawberries	1 large pancake, 4 sausage links, 2 tsp butter, 2 Tbs syrup, 1 cup of strawberries
Breakfast 3	2 pieces of multigrain bread, 3 slices of turkey bacon, ½ tomato sliced, 2 tsp mayo	1 piece of multigrain bread, 6 slices of turkey bacon, ½ tomato sliced, 2 tsp mayo, orange slices
	Weight Maintenance 2:1	*Metabolic Balance 1:1*
Morning snack 1	1 cup 4% cottage cheese, 1 cup cut pineapple	½ cup 4% cottage cheese, 1 cup cut pineapple
Morning snack 2	2 hard-boiled eggs, 1 small cranberry nut roll	1 hard-boiled egg, 1 small cranberry nut roll
Morning snack 3	6 pieces of celery with 2 Tbs almond butter	6 pieces of celery with 1 Tbs almond butter

Table 6.3 Food Log: Metabolic Balance, Morning

Event Time	Event	Pre EE Intention	Food Consumed	C	P	F	F/V	Hunger/ Fullness (Before/ After)	Pacing: Fast (F) Moderate (M) Slow (S)	Symptoms	What I Noticed	What's Next Intention	Action Plan
6:30 am	Woke up												
07:30	Breakfast	Eat a balanced meal	Bacon, egg, and cheese on bagel	O	A	A	U	2/8	M	Unbalanced	I remember feeling like an egg sandwich would not be enough. I noticed the chewy bagel	Be mindful of meal plan	Tomorrow get egg and cheese sandwich with tomato
09:30	Snack		Blueberry muffin	O	–	O	–	4/7	F	Unplanned	Checked out		
10:30	Snack		10 Hershey Kisses	–	–	O	–	4/7	F	Compulsive eating/binge	Once I started I couldn't stop. I noticed I wanted to keep taste going in my mouth. I noticed the mouthfeel of chocolate	Practice stopping the symptom	Mindful Awareness break: 1) 5 breaths 2) check in with body, emotions, thoughts 3) distract with Iphone game for 15 minutes 4) check in again. 5) Go back to class

The breath exercise has two steps: inhale while lifting the shoulders slightly, and then exhale through an open mouth while letting go of the shoulders (depressing them down). I also made sure to explain the science behind his body's reaction to anxiety:

> When you are anxious, your sympathetic nervous system (SNS) is heightened, putting you in fight, flight, or freeze mode. Our body is designed that way for a good reason; a quickly activated SNS stimulates your body to secrete a slew of hormones to help us avoid getting hit by a bus or (in the old days) eaten by a bear. To hurl us into "fight, flight, or freeze" action, the hormones:
>
> - make it difficult to eat
> - shunt blood away from the gut to our peripheral extremities, like legs and arms
> - biologically blunt our hunger cues
> - stimulate hyper-awareness
> - stifle appetite.
>
> The way your body operates, your SNS can't tell if "activation" is triggered by a bus, a bear, or a breakfast. But we can deal with that.
>
> Fortunately, your *pranayama* practice is your new superpower: the ability to calm your SNS and your body through the power of breath.

We practiced the breath exercise several times in my office over a couple of appointments. He eventually reported that *pranayama* was especially helpful to use while waking up, getting ready for school, and eating breakfast.

This chapter's meal plans and food logs represent a client working toward metabolic balance (Tables 6.2 and 6.3).

Midday

We already know that midday brings a crescendo of signals that stimulate anxiety and stress in people with eating disorders. It feels like data overload and, rather than steam coming out of their ears, they react with symptom thoughts and behaviors of every variety.

At the same time, the crescendo contains plenty of data to notice, collect, and categorize. This is a good thing!

Consider a patient approaching lunch. We ask:

1. What do you notice about your body's fullness/hunger level right now?
2. What do you notice about how your body is reacting or responding (physiologically) to its fullness/hunger level?

3.   Do you notice any thoughts or emotions?
4.   What do you think it might mean that you:

   a.   can notice your body's fullness/hunger level right now?
   b.   can't notice your body's fullness/hunger level right now?
   c.   have trouble noticing your body's fullness/hunger level right now?

One of my patients has anxiety that blunts hunger and fullness cues. In response, we developed midday noticing practice. She stops every day at 12:30 to do a mindful scan of her body and notice what is happening.

•   Notice your breath right now. What can you notice about it?
•   Notice your body sensations right now. Tell me what you notice about them.
•   Notice your thoughts in this moment. What is the energy around your thoughts?
•   Notice feelings or emotions present. What can you notice about their intensity?
•   What does your noticing data tell you?

She identified mental fogginess, low energy, and increased anxiety in her body. We guide her to associate (she calls it "syncing up") those sensations with her body's midday needs and cues. The practice dramatically reduced her lunch anxiety and resistance. She labeled fogginess, low energy, and increased anxiety as simple, matter-of-fact signals for: "It's lunch time. It's time to eat."

She continued observing these cues over time, and the practice generated more frequent sensations of being in her body. Now she's starting to notice physiological hunger cues at midday. That's important recovery growth, clearing the path between her and her body.

Mindful practice can happen in any environment. For example, one of my meal coaches took a client to a busy food court for lunch. Because the client was terrified to eat with so much external stimulation, they started with a pre-meal awareness check:

•   Notice your breath right now. What do you notice about it?
•   Notice your body right now. Tell me what you notice about it.
•   What do you notice about your degree of hunger?
•   Notice your thoughts and feelings right now. What are they?
•   What intention can you set for the next five minutes?

They walked together to each food stand before considering what foods to eat. Then they did another mindful check. Next, they decided on the food, ordered and got their meals, and sat at a table. They did more mindful checks before, during, and after the meal. A patient's "new" data helps them notice the arc of sensations during eating events.

Noticing data also informs patients as they practice creating intentions. For example, we use these prompts in a meal support group:

- Set an intention for this meal before you start. Then, share your intention with me/us.
- Set an intention for interacting with the other people in the group while you eat.
- As the meals ends, check in on your intention, and share what you noticed with me/us.
- Set an intention for the time period after this meal and share it with me/us.
- (Before the next eating event begins) Check in on your last "after the meal" intention and share and/or journal what you noticed.

Before and after intentions and/or action plans help patients manage their sensations. Here are a few action plans from my former patients:

- I feel so full right now, but my action step is to go home and have a snack before bed.
- I know it is really important for me to journal when I get home, because that's when I would want to purge.
- I will remind myself tonight that I will follow my plan tomorrow.
- I need to walk a little bit in order to make it through the rest of the day, but I won't over-exercise. Instead, I'll get off the subway one stop early and walk home the extra 10 blocks.
- My girlfriend and I will walk the dog right after dinner, so I stay out of the bathroom and out of the house while my urges lessen and/or pass.

The data helps them notice the arc of their sensations (physical and emotional) throughout the day. The data informs intentions for the time period between now and the next eating event. For example: "How do I want to experience the next three hours until my mini-meal?"

We invite them to choose an intention by answering simple questions like:

- How do I want my experience of this meal to go?
- What do I want to work on with this meal?
- How do I want to pace the eating?
- What do I want to receive from this meal?
- What do I want to receive during this meal?

We hear a wide range of intentions during Mindful Eating. Most of them are concrete and accomplishable:

- I want to stay present to the meal, so I can eat in a moderate way.
- When I feel really scared of a food, I will eat to get through it anyway.
- I want to enjoy the meal and try to get my thoughts and feelings out of the way so I can do that.
- I want to eat more slowly.
- I want to eat more mindfully.
- I just want to get through the damn thing!

Even intentions born of frustration and impatience are important, because that means the person is using their newfound "noticing" data and new-found skills to "notice" how they get through that damned meal!

Table 6.4 Meal Plan, Midday

	Weight Maintenance 2:1:1:1	*Metabolic Balance 1:2:1:2*
Lunch 1	Sandwich on 2 slices rye made with deli turkey (3 oz), ⅛th avocado, lettuce, tomato	Sandwich on English muffin with deli turkey (6 oz), ⅛th avocado, lettuce, tomato, and 1 cup of baby carrots
Lunch 2	2 California rolls, side salad with ginger dressing	1 California roll, side salad with ginger dressing, 4 pieces of sashimi
Lunch 3	2 pieces of bbq chicken, side of mac and cheese	3 pieces of bbq chicken, 1 biscuit
	Weight Maintenance 1:1:1:1	*Metabolic Balance 0.5:1:1:1*
Mini-meal 1	½ cup vegetable lentil soup, 2 breadsticks with 2 tsp butter	½ cup vegetable lentil soup, 1 breadstick with 2 tsp butter
Mini-meal 2	1 serving of tortilla chips, 1 oz of shredded cheese, 1 Tbs sour cream, jalepeño peppers	½ serving of tortilla chips, 1 oz of shredded cheese, 1 Tbs sour cream, jalepeño peppers
Mini-meal 3	2 small pitas with ¼ cup hummus, 2 Tbs baba ganoush	1 small pita with ¼ cup hummus, 2 Tbs baba ganoush
	Weight Maintenance 2:1	*Metabolic Balance 1:1*
Late-afternoon snack	1/4 cup almonds, serving of dried apricots	2 Tbs almonds, one serving of dried apricots
Late-afternoon snack	1 sheet of Graham crackers, 8 oz of kefir	1 sheet of Graham crackers, 4 oz of kefir
Late-afternoon snack	1 serving of potato chips, 2 string cheese	1 serving of potato chips, 1 string cheese

Table 6.5 Food Log: Metabolic Balance, Midday

Event Time	Event	Pre EIE Intention	Food Consumed	C	P	F	F/V	Hunger/ Fullness (Before/ After)	Pacing: Fast (F) Moderate (M) Slow (S)	Symptoms	What I Noticed	What's Next Intention	Action Plan
13:30	Lunch	Practice mindfulness	3 Jamaican beef patties, lemonade	O	A	A	A	3/8	M	Overate	I noticed I as eating very fast	Bring awareness into the day	Plan snack now for later: Kind bar, grapes
04:30	Mini-meal		Kind bar, grapes	A	A	A	A	3/6	F	None	I noticed the sweetness of chocolate, savory flavor of peanuts, juice grapes	Stay on track!	Plan dinner now! Shop and cook dinner at home

The meal plan and food log in Tables 6.4 and 6.5 represent a client working toward metabolic balance.

Late in the Day

Daytime routines and responsibilities provide an outlet for perfectionism. Indeed, some employers and teachers value the person's hyper-responsibility as evidence of productivity. As they practice mindfulness, many patients notice that the structure, predictability, and expectations of their daytime routines and responsibilities act as containers. Ironically, they also give the eating disorder predictable moments to hijack the authentic self.

What happens when they leave daytime routines and responsibilities? People with eating disorders often feel less safe. Because eating disorders thrive in both predictability and uncertainty, it's "safe" either way.

As our patients head back to homes, apartments, and dorms, they usually have a mishmash of feelings and thoughts. "If my daytime eating leaves my body malnourished, I probably won't have energy or focus to manage at-home mishmash without my symptoms."

Whether nourished or not, the body slows down in the evening, guiding our brains and bodies into a fruitful, vulnerable state for noticing and processing emotions. We're likely to laugh and cry our hardest late in the day.

Therefore, when our patients practice noticing, they need skills to cope with and manage what they notice.

Table 6.6 Meal Plan, Evening

	Weight Maintenance 2:1:1:1	*Metabolic Balance 1:2:1:2*
Dinner 1	Turkey burger on bun, small side salad with dressing, ½ serving of fries	Turkey burger on bun, small side salad with dressing
Dinner 2	Tofu stir fry with 1 cup of brown rice and 1 cup of vegetables	Tofu stir fry with ½ cup of brown rice and 2 cups of vegetables
Dinner 3	3 oz broiled cod fish, 2 cobs of corn, 1 cup broiled cauliflower	6oz broiled cod fish, 1 cob of corn, 1½ cups broiled cauliflower
	Weight Maintenance 2:1	*Metabolic Balance 1:1*
Evening snack 1	½ cup ricotta with vanilla and cinnamon sugar on 1 piece cinnamon raisin bread	¼ cup ricotta with vanilla and cinnamon sugar on 1 piece cinnamon raisin bread
Evening snack 2	½ cup of overnight oats made with milk, topped with ½ cup Greek yogurt	½ cup of overnight oats made with milk
Evening snack 3	6 pieces of pepperoni, 1 serving of Ritz crackers	3 pieces of pepperoni, 1 serving of Ritz crackers

Table 6.7 Food Log: Metabolic Balance, Evening

Event Time	Event	Pre EE Intention	Food Consumed	C	P	F	F/V	Hunger/ Fullness (Before/ After)	Pacing: Fast (F) Moderate (M) Slow (S)	Symptoms	What I Noticed	What's Next Intention	Action Plan
18:00	30– minute walk home from campus	Move my body!									Felt hard to be in my body at first but then I felt strong	Do this more often!	
8:00 pm	Dinner	Determined to have balanced meal	Large piece of catfish, ¼ cup mashed pota- toes, 2 cups of collards	A	A	A	A	3/8	M	No!	What I noticed most was my sense of pride of making this meal	Manage overeating urges	Go to bed
10:45	Snack	End the day off right	2 handfuls of trail mix	–	A	A	A	3/5	M	No!	I noticed the sweet and savory flavors. I noticed the small parts between my fingers. I also noticed I was tired	Remember to pack this snack for tomor- row to bring to school when I want some- thing snack on	

One of our patients is a teacher. Upon entering the house around 4:00, they stand in front of the refrigerator with their coat on, rummage through the shelves, and eat mindlessly. They recognize this as a disconnected experience, but say it is how they know they are home and not in school any more.

During the six weeks another client waited to hear about a promotion, she reported: "Every night, I'm consumed with 'moving at the speed of light' thoughts about my meetings, emails, projects, boss, and on and on. Eating is the furthest thing from my mind." Only after her husband came home did she notice she'd been stuck for hours in a loop of obsessive, anxious thoughts.

We respond by teaching each patient skills for mindful acceptance. We make sure to dispel the myth that acceptance equals resignation and/or defeat ("I give up; I'll just have to live with the fear and pain"). We (repeatedly) redefine acceptance as the *practice* of using awareness to deepen compassion in the moment. One skill is practicing (repeatedly) acceptance self-talk.

- I can't feel my hunger cues because I am anxious right now. But I know my body needs food right now.
- My eating disorder is telling me I can hold out another few hours. My body is telling me it's tired. I know "tired" is another way to understand when to eat my snack and give my body the energy it needs right now.
- I ate dinner and (not but!) I am still feeling hungry. I want more food, but I know and trust that the amount on my meal plan is what my body needs today. So, I will tolerate wanting more food until I fall asleep.
- I want a chocolate sundae, but I understand it will make me feel queasy if I eat it right now. I will eat my mini-meal in 15 minutes and then, if I still want ice cream later, I can add it to my dinner.
- I wish I didn't like this meal so much. It's scary to like it this much. But I can enjoy the taste right now.

When clients learn to shine the light of awareness on what is (e.g., juggling two balls), it steadily increases their ability to accept what they notice about food, feeding, and body. Practicing acceptance paves the way for a deeper sense of knowing and trusting that our body *does* know. Developing these skills naturally leads to Intuitive Eating and stronger recovery.

Resisting Gravitational Pull

For many of our patients, the relationship with the eating disorder is the most central relationship in life.

It's as if the disorder is a sun creating its solar system out of a person's thoughts, emotional reactions, behaviors, other relationships, and spirit. The longer these "planets" revolve around the eating disorder, the more stubborn its gravitational pull.

Drawing any of those "planets" away and into recovery star's orbit takes enormous energy. However, each time a planet breaks free, the disorder's gravitational power diminishes.

The journey of recovery can feel like defying universal laws of physics. Awareness taps a life force energy with enough power to pull the self into a new and authentic orbit.

Our clinicians use "mindful moments" to help patient stay present in the now, and plan for staying present during the rest of the day. Here's an example:

THEM: I don't know how to schedule the rest of my day with food.

ME: Tell me more. How did your day go?

THEM: I got into work at 8:30 and had a meeting at 9:00.

ME: Breakfast?

THEM: Well they had coffee and muffins, so I ate one around 9:30.

ME: What did you notice about your energy level?

THEM: I felt OK but by the time the meeting was over I was starving and tired.

ME: OK. That's why it's so important to balance your meal when you can. Then what happened?

THEM: Well, I missed my snack, so I ate an early lunch. I had pork tacos and a side of beans.

ME: Do you remember how you felt after you ate lunch?

THEM: I felt great. I guess that's what you meant about balancing, huh?

ME: Yep, that's exactly what I meant.

THEM: I started feeling hungry around 2:30, but then my girlfriend called, and we got into a fight. I got upset, so I wasn't hungry any more. I didn't have a snack and then I had to run out to get to this appointment.

ME: How do you feel now?

THEM: I don't know, upset.

ME: Where in your body do you feel upset?

THEM: My stomach is turning.

ME: OK. Could it be that your emotions are taking up space in your belly, so you're not going to feel your hunger? You still need to eat that mini-meal as soon as you leave here. Then dinner four hours later. And even if you're still not feeling your hunger, you need to plan a balanced snack before bed.

THEM: OK, I get it. It's not going to be easy to eat when I'm not hungry, but I know my body needs the food.

Through two Mindful Eating chapters, we've yet to encounter any Buddhist monks sitting cross-legged in the Himalayan snow (or drinking tea).

Mindfulness is simultaneously simple, tricky, challenging, and taxing. We as clinicians—and our patients as individuals—must dive headfirst into the container we call the body. We help our clients reclaim (and then protect) their "homes" from invasions. We advocate for them and their bodies—inviting them to treat themselves like precious children.

We clinicians may (or will) feel tempted to skip over or speed up this edgy phase. Then, we remember how much it delivers. Mindful Eating is an amazing springboard into the new. With it, we guide the people in our care toward new suns to orbit.

Bibliography

Ackerman, D. *A Natural History of the Senses* (New York: Vintage, 1990).

Katzman, D.K., Norris, M.L., and Zucker, N. (2019). Avoidant restrictive food intake disorder. *Psychiatric Clinics of North America*, 42, 1.

7 Intuitive Eating

Intuition is difficult to define, yet we know it's more than a thinking process. Yoga tradition says the seat of intuition is in the body. In a quiet mind, we can move into deeper parts of the body, access our inner wisdom, and experience intuition. Spiritual and yoga practice "quiet" the mind, slow down thoughts, and pause reactivity.

Advances in neuroscience (including fMRI) illustrate that breathing, meditation, and posture-based yoga increase overall brain wave activity, along with amygdala and frontal cortex activation. Some researchers find signs that yoga may also beneficially change brain physiology and structures.

Intuitive Eating invites and prompts clients to take risks that feel different than what they've risked so far in recovery. Clients step farther away from prescriptive eating, their treatment team, and their eating disorder identity. They step closer to relationships that don't revolve around eating disorders. That territory is unfamiliar, less predictable, and more fluid. Most of them still butt heads with symptoms, while slowing down to discern, decide, and determine what to do next. The experience can feel liberating and flexible, frightening and volatile, or all of the above all at the same time.

People in our care open safe paths to their "inner eater" and inner wisdom. This facilitates freedom in relationships with self, body, and eating disorder. The paths then begin to cross bridges into the wide world of vital and imperfect relationships with themselves, other people, creativity, spirituality, recreation, vocation, and more.

Most clients experience this phase as a major leap toward recovery.

Taking the Wheel

People can take months or years to explore and integrate Intuitive Eating and all its nuances. Fortunately, during Intuitive Eating, clients often feel the same kind of excitement, thrill, and anxiety we had the first time we got in a car to drive. They practice with a clinician "driving instructor" in the passenger seat.

Before putting the car in gear, the not-ready-for-road-time driver must learn lots of data and patterns from the driving instructor, state driver's manual, and the vehicle owner's manual. Once behind the wheel, the student driver goes slowly while the driving instructor guides, coaches, points out mistakes, points out danger spots, and suggests safe tactics and timing. They say things like: "Look in the rearview mirror regularly, but not for long; it's more important to keep your eyes on the road ahead."

The instructor must have patience and be willing to repeat everything they say, because the student driver is overloaded with sensory and memory data. Student and instructor must practice the granular and big-picture skills, often simultaneously. Student and instructor must also have tolerance for risk, since the student is (in real time and real traffic) trying to process information, apply it to as-yet-theoretical patterns of driving, and not hurt anyone.

Can you recall the tension, fear, and frustration you felt while first learning to drive? Do you recall feeling impatient because your driving instructor (and/or parents) made you wait before giving you the car keys? Do you recall the fear and/or cockiness you had as a new driver, and how you overcame it? Do you recall the freedom and flexibility driving gave you?

Finally, when was the last time we thought about learning to drive? Today, it feels like a minuscule blip on the map of life, even as we continue our driving "practice" every day.

During recovery, we clinicians remind ourselves and our clients of the real or potential forward movement in every session, meal, log entry, and email. During Intuitive Eating, we aim to give clients the wheel and begin driving their own recovery.

Recovery radically increases freedom. A recovered friend describes it this way:

> I have the experience now. I can face uncertainty without letting fear paralyze me. In fact, if I keep practicing, I feel energized, calm, and joyful at the same time!
>
> When it comes to eating, I know what's going to happen. Like if you've eaten pizza a thousand times, fear may pop up on the 1,001st time. But I can look back and say, "As of today, a slice of pizza has never done what my eating disorder told me it was going to do." That was true the first time, the second time, the third time—even when I believed the eating disorder's lies about pizza and every other food. My recovery actions and understanding and attitudes give me proof that I can trust my choice to eat *this* pizza in *this* moment. I can trust my body to use it wisely. I love getting to a place where I can respect my body's wisdom. I definitely think the payoff is freedom.

A Bit of Context

Our practice's intake process always asks: "What is your goal?" Many clients reply: "I want to learn how to eat intuitively." When we ask them to tell us more, their answers boil down to desires like these: "I want to develop more freedom. I want to keep eating disorder thoughts from gripping my mind. I want symptoms to stop invading my eating."

Evelyn Tribole and Elyse Resch's 1995 book *Intuitive Eating* had a huge impact on our nutrition field. It filled a glaring gap. Rooted in an anti-diet movement, their approach helps people to practice letting go of judgmental thoughts about food and our body, while learning to listen to the body's inner cues. They issued a clear call to adopt a food-neutral perspective and stop seeing foods as "bad/unhealthy" or "good/healthy." They encouraged people to take their cravings, preferences, and hunger signals seriously.

They vividly illustrated how the body intuitively knows its need for balanced and timely nutrition. The body can get balanced and timely nutrition from a wide variety of foods. Therefore, we can trust our bodies and be flexible eaters. Tribole and Resch use the memorable image of someone eating the same food at every meal every day. All other things being equal, the person's body will eventually make clear that this narrow approach doesn't work—no matter if the food is chocolate cake or organic spinach.

The book remains a game changer for countless people (me included).

Not surprisingly, clinicians treating eating disorders found valuable concepts and tools in *Intuitive Eating*. Its ideas continue to inform our ongoing inquiry into the full spectrum of eating disorders, how to care for them effectively, and what's missing in our approaches to recovery.

However, even Tribole and Resch recognize that, without significant alteration, a trust-your-body approach proves problematic for people with active eating disorders. After all, is it safe to trust a disordered, dysregulated, malnourished body?

Consider a person with active anorexia who restricts all day, and then "listens" for body signals. The signals include loud and abusive eating disorder messages. But the person's blunted hunger cues won't get through. The result of this listening? The person hears "don't eat," continues restricting, and keeps endangering their body.

Now, consider a person with active binge eating disorder. Hearing that there are no "bad" foods, they might eat brownies for dinner every day for months. The person's metabolism is dangerously out of balance. However, the eating disorder blocks the metabolism's "Help me, I need other stuff!" signals. The person doesn't hear: "It's time for balanced eating" when listening to their disordered, dysregulated, malnourished body. They hear: "I want to eat brownies for 100 *more* days."

The most recovery-committed patients can lose ground if they attempt to "follow their gut" while their hunger and satiety cues remain misaligned and out of sync with body processes. In recovery, Intuitive Eating is a highly attuned, advanced skill.

Fortunately, clients and their experience never stop teaching eating disorder professionals which treatment elements work and which ones don't. Recovery-informed Intuitive Eating practices are critical recovery skills.

Where We're Headed

On the first day of my nutrition science master's program, the professor said: "When it comes to nutrition, there's only one thing people need to know: variety is how people survive on this planet." I am a *Homo sapiens* who lives on Long Island, with easy access to beef and fish—but not yak. Some *Homo sapiens* live where they have easy access to yak, but not beef or fish. Some live where they don't have access to animal protein, but do have access to legumes and rice, a combination that delivers complete proteins, with the same amino acids as beef or yak.

Our species still exists because our bodies are capable of getting the nutrition they need from many different foods. No one had to move people from Tibet to Cuba to get the "right" foods. No tech entrepreneur invented this capacity. Our bodies did.

The bodies of people with eating disorders often lose connection to this basic scientific fact. Our bodies have a superpower: they can create or recreate the nutrition knowledge and flexibility inherent in our species. Here's how I explain it to patients:

> Our body can identify and use every food we've ever consumed, or ever will consume. Imagine every protein, carbohydrate, fat, and fruit/vegetable that entered your body, from mother's milk to today's banana. Now imagine that:
>
> • Your body knew how to use every one of them.
> • Your body still knows; every food you eat leaves an imprint behind.

When a body is nutritionally aligned, it senses the substances it needs. You don't consciously realize that your body currently needs lysine, tryptophan, alpha-linolenic acid, eicosapentaenoic acid, docosahexaenoic acid, niacin, thiamine, iron, or phosphorus. Instead, you feel a hankering for salmon with spinach (which contain all those nutrients with long names). You are intuiting that salmon and spinach work for you right now.

In other words, our bodies already know the answers. Intuitive Eating teaches us how to hear and follow what our bodies (and our spirits) know. That is pretty basic—and very cool.

Your body knew this all along, but your path to the knowledge was buried under a whole bunch of other things—like eating disorder symptoms and patterns. We have to clear symptoms from the path before we can connect to wise, fact-based dialogues between you and the body. We're working on that now during Intuitive Eating.

We're entering an exciting time when clients start talking about more than food: relationships, personal environment, wellbeing, and so on. When talk does turns to food, conversations are driven by curiosity and understanding. Clients are learning to trust and make more room to have a dialogue with authentic and spiritual parts of themselves.

Of course, patients also say, "This might be exciting for you, but it's scary as s*** for me right now." We acknowledge that the nutritionist must still hold the excitement when the patient holds the fear. Other times, the patient holds the excitement and the nutritionist holds caution and/or fear. Intuitive

Eating is rich with relational aspects. One is the clinician and the patient trusting each other on the way to exciting and scary autonomy.

Clients make this exciting recovery leap by practicing discernment, differentiation, learning from their edges and patterns, choice, decisions, and discovering preferences.

Discernment

Patients notice and gather a lot of data during Mindful Eating. They transition to Intuitive Eating by layering on discernment: the process of clarifying the collected information. From there, they can notice and identify new or existing patterns. They can notice and identify ways their data relates to and influences other data. They can notice and identify ways data relates to and influences their patterns. They can notice and identify ways their patterns relate to and influence each other.

We start by practicing differentiating between "physical hunger and fullness" and "emotional hunger and fullness." Of course, emotions are in the body; the physical/emotional terminology is shorthand for the digestive function and nutrient absorption (physical) and limbic system information (emotional).

When your body needs hydration, you can easily recognize "Oh, I'm thirsty" and drink a glass of water. Our water-hunger stimulus and response might not be fully conscious. But they usually have a clear communication channel. It's open and easy because we recognize the physical locations of our thirst sensations: dry mouth, tongue, or throat; lightheaded head, and so on.

Emotional hunger and fullness are more difficult to discern. We can feel lost and uncertain during floods of emotion, numbed emotions, confused emotions, and so forth. The difficulty increases exponentially when you have an eating disorder and/or another mental illness, like posttraumatic stress disorder (PTSD), depression, anxiety, addiction, etc., which many people with eating disorders have.

We use several techniques to help clients practice this discernment. Our Intuitive Eating food log includes familiar items from previous phases, and adds two new categories:

1   who I ate with/where I ate
2   emotional hunger/fullness; the scale is 0 = numbed, 1 = under-stimulated, 2 = slight feeling, 3 = mild feeling, 4 = neutral feeling, 5 = adequate feeling, 6 = moderate feeling, 7 = strong feeling, 8 = intense feeling, 9 = over-stimulated, 10 = flooded.

We use that data to ask deeper questions and dig into what sensations prompted them to use the numbers in the scales. Table 7.1 shows an Intuitive Eating weight maintenance food log:

Table 7.1 Food Log: Weight Maintenance, All Day

Event Time	Event	Who I Ate With/Where I Ate	Movement/Activity/Exercise	Pre EE Intention	Food Consumed	Physical Hunger/Fullness (Before/After)	Emotional Hunger/Fullness	Pacing: Fast (F) Moderate (M) Slow (S)	Symptoms	What I Noticed	What's Next Intention	Action Plan
6:15 am	Wake up											
06:45	Breakfast	At home, getting kids breakfast and myself	Making beds, getting kids ready	Even though I'm multi-tasking I want to stay aware of what I'm eating	Toasted mini-bagel, with smear of cream cheese and 2 pieces of smoked salmon, sliced tomato, a few bites of kids' left-over eggs	2/6	6/5	M	NA	I am noticing how much more comfortable I am with eating bagels now than a year ago. I love bagels!		
07:45	Exercise		Vinyasa flow class				3			Ohmmm. Very relaxed, feel good in my body. Strong and confident		

10:00	Myself at yoga studio/smoothie bar	Feed my body after moving it	Medium smoothie with berries, soy-milk, and banana	3/6	4/5	M	NA	I noticed other people with smaller bodies not getting smoothies	Keep my focus on my body and its needs	To be a zen master in recovery one must drink their smoothie. Take five full breaths
1:30 pm	Applebees with Sue	Listen to my body when making lunch choice, was craving red meat	Burger with cheddar, salad with dressing	2/8	7/8	F	Speedy eating	Was nice to connect with Sue. I noticed a bit of social anxiety. I noticed I was eating fast as a result. I had a craving for a burger. I'm getting my period soon! *Need iron stat*	Stay in my body and move through anxiety	
14:00	5-minute awareness break	Just checking in with my body		5	6			I noticed I still feeling a bit anxious. I noticed tightness in my chest, breathing a bit shallow, thoughts racing on my never-ending to-do list	Take a step back	Make a to-do list. Pack with me for snack. Remind myself I am enough without having to produce. Know it'll be OK

(Continued)

Table 7.1 (Cont.)

Event Time	Event	Who I Ate With/ Where I Ate	Move- ment/ Activity/ Exercise	Pre EE Intention	Food Consumed	Physical Hunger/ Fullness (Before/ After)	Emotional Hunger/ Fullness	Pacing: Fast (F) Moderate (M) Slow (S)	Symptoms	What I Noticed	What's Next Intention	Action Plan
5:00 pm	Mini- meal	In the car, with kids, soccer practice		Making myself impor- tant!	2 cheese sticks, pack of pretzels, handful of grapes	4/6	6/6	M		Feel proud that I took five minutes to grab this snack along with soccer gear, water bottles, and snacks for kids	Gratitude	Pat myself on the back… literally
07:30	Dinner	Table, family	Does making dinner, setting table, and washing dishes count? LOL	Eat with inten- tion but intui- tively	Chicken stir fry with rice and vegetables. Had 1 large bowl then checked in with hunger and had another small helping	3/7	7/6	M				

Time											
7:50 pm	Dessert	Washing dinner		Honor my craving	Piece of dark chocolate	7/8	4/5	S	I wanted something sweet. I am still full from dinner. I thoroughly enjoyed this piece of chocolate. It was yummy and hit the spot. It was exactly what I wanted	Bedtime is always a little harried. I'm making the intention to find a balance between getting things done but staying in my body	Had a conversation with my spouse. Told them I needed their support to get evening tasks done
10:30 pm	Snack	In kitchen, at table myself	Crawling up to bed	Notice my exhaustion	Cup of cereal with milk	3/6	9/0	M	I'm a bit checked out. I'm really tired and still feel a part of my brain on overdrive	Take it down a notch	Hot shower
11:05 pm	Sleep										

Here's what the nutritionist and clients are looking for in each column:

- Event time: helps us know where they are in the day and where they will be next. They plan eating events accordingly.
- Event: waking, sleeping, eating events, and other notable daily events.
- Who I ate with/where I ate: helps patient and provider discern *environment* patterns such as: I eat all my meals by myself, I eat at my desk a lot, I need to consider not eating in front of the TV.
- Movement/activity/exercise: helps patient and provider see frequency and intensity patterns in physical activity, how the patterns support recovery, and whether they are symptoms or veering close to symptomatic.
- Pre EE (eating event) intention: practice focusing recovery-driven energy on to the next eating activity.
- Food consumed: what and about how much.
- Physical hunger/fullness (before/after): practice discerning the body's physiological cues.
- Emotional hunger/fullness: practice discerning the body's emotional and relational cues.
- Pacing: fast (F), moderate (M), slow (S): helps patient and provider discern pacing pattern, and how they relate to eating environment, physiological cues, emotional and relational cues, etc.
- Symptoms: tracks symptom use particular to this day and time of the day when symptom occurred. Helps patient and provider understand longer-term patterns and triggers.
- What I noticed: an "abbreviated" mindfulness journal to help patient and provider discern and discuss patterns.
- What's next intention: helps patient to consider how to continue their recovery eating path or make important intentions to alter patterns that block and detour the path.
- Action plan: prompts patient to decide on concrete actions that help them move forward into the next part of the day.

With practice, people accurately sense evidence that their *eating* fullness level is 0, 5, 10, or somewhere in between. That facilitates the practice of using physical sensations to identify whether *other* fullness levels (emotional, relational, etc.) are 0, 5, 10, or somewhere in between.

Yoga-informed nutrition helps clients discern what their sensations are communicating.

CLIENT: I'm feeling really full.
CLINICIAN: Can you tell me where in your body that feeling is? And can you describe the sensations you're having there?
CLIENT: I'm feeling pressure and discomfort in my belly.
CLINICIAN: OK. When did you eat last and what did you have?

CLIENT: I finished lunch around a half-hour ago. I had a tuna fish sandwich with lettuce and tomato and ate an orange afterward.

CLINICIAN: Does that seem like enough food to give your body what it needs for the next few hours? Does it feel like too much?

CLIENT: I think it's about the right amount.

CLINICIAN: OK. That's good data to include. Let's go back to your belly now.

CLIENT: Ugh. That just makes me wanna puke. But, OK.

CLINICIAN: What are you picking up about your sensations now?

CLIENT: Well, I'm still feeling pressure, like I ate too much. But it doesn't make sense for that to be food hunger.

CLINICIAN: OK. Let me ask what's been happening in the rest of your life since yesterday.

CLIENT: Well, my boss has been hypercritical, and it's upsetting and making me tense.

CLINICIAN: Where is the feeling of upset hanging out in your body?

CLIENT: In my belly.

CLINICIAN: Do you think the sensations of upset and feeling like you ate too much have any connection?

CLIENT: I'm not sure. I just know I feel overwhelmed. I don't know what to do. When my boss is breathing down my neck, it's too much for me.

CLINICIAN: Can you identify ways that belly-related things, like eating, purging, nausea, etc. relate to upset for you? Do they ever provide a solution or give you any useful information?

CLIENT: Well, I know enough to know that purging isn't really a solution any more. And I guess that my stomach is telling me I'm on emotional overload, and I feel stuffed and stuck. That's no solution.

CLINICIAN: True. And now you've discerned that your "stuffed-ness" is emotional. Purging isn't going to help us get closer to what this emotion is really about. And that's where my nutritionist job ends, and your therapist's job picks up.

CLIENT: Oh great, so now I've discerned the problem and you're telling me that you're passing the buck? You're depriving me of a solution? You're abandoning me?

CLINICIAN: I hear you. And I'm not going anywhere. I'm staying in my "lane" and working with you from my knowledge, just as your therapist works from their knowledge. And we will keep working together on it.

The conversation illustrates the need to help the people in our care recognize a variety of fullness/hunger situations, for example:

- I can eat a half of a sandwich and be emotionally full but still physically hungry.

- I can eat two sandwiches and be physically overfull but emotionally empty.
- I can eat one sandwich and feel emotionally satisfied and physically satisfied.
- I can eat a half of a sandwich and be emotionally hungry and physically hungry.
- I can eat two sandwiches and be physically overfull and emotionally over-stuffed.
- I can eat one sandwich and feel emotionally empty and still a little hungry physically.
- And so on.

Practicing discernment helps clients pick up:

- Psychological cues, like thoughts that interrupt and intrude upon the physiologic system. "I know it's time to eat but my eating disorder voice is telling me that I shouldn't."
- Relational cues, like the actions of people around us. "Everybody else is still dancing, but I sense my body saying that it's hungry right now."
- Emotional cues, like elation over a situation or experience. "My brother is married! I truly can join my family's love and joy while we all eat wedding cake and drink champagne together!"
- Simultaneous, contrasting cues, like eating a satisfying dinner with friends, and then going to a movie theater where the friends buy popcorn to share. "I'm not physically hungry at the moment. But the popcorn smells good. It's easy for me to eat popcorn mindlessly. What do I want to do next?"

The cues aren't always clear, of course. Here's how one of my yoga therapy clients described learning to discern: "It's like when you're trying to communicate with someone when you speak English and they speak French but you both know a little bit of Spanish."

Remember Table 1.1 in Chapter 1, comparing disordered and fulfilling human relationships? It can help clients discern relational, emotional, and psychological satiety. We reproduced it here as Table 7.2 with different headings.

Drawing on Dr. Margo Maine's groundbreaking work in *Father Hunger: Fathers, Daughters and Food*, my co-author Joe Kelly (author of *Dads and Daughters*) uses these questions when working with adult daughters:

- What do I hunger for, seek, want, desire, etc. from my father and/or stepfather?
- How reasonable is it to expect that this hunger will be fed by relationships with my father and/or stepfather?

Table 7.2 Types of Human Relationships

Under- and Over-Filled Human Relationships	Fulfilling Human Relationships
Hide and deny needs for emotional, relational, spiritual (etc.) connection	Feed your natural human hungers for connection, meaning, comfort, etc.
Avoid new or different people; maintaining contact with very few people	Inviting and being involved with people and situations that are truly and mutually fulfilling
End for fear of difficult emotions, other people's opinions, cultural constructs	Do not end just because someone or something else disapproves
Hide and deny needs for emotional, relational, spiritual (etc.) connection. Try to control the other person's behavior	Dedicate thought and intention while inviting and deepening your relationship, so you are nourished spiritually, emotionally, psychologically, etc.
Judgmental, rigid, and fear-filled rules about other people and relationships	Enjoying and embracing people and situations different from what you are used to
Blame others for how I feel. Try to control the other person's behavior	Give yourself permission to be together with another person sometimes because you are happy, sad, bored, or just because it feels good
Feel abandoned by others. Resent and try to control the other person's behavior	Can mean being together occasionally, regularly, and/or nearly all the time
Feel smothered by others. Resent and try to control the other person's behavior	Can survive overload, recognizing the need for autonomy and occasional time away from one another
Feel abandoned by others. Resent and try to control the other person's behavior	Can survive separation, recognizing how absence makes the heart grow fonder
Hide and deny thoughts and feelings. Try to control the other person's behavior	Develops instincts and intuition; trusting your emotions, sensations, and wisdom, etc.
Focus all/most attention on trying to control the other person's behavior	Take time and attention, but is not the only important area of your life

- What other relationships and/or experiences might feed my father hunger?

We can use or adapt tools like this to help people in our care recognize—and embody—how their relational hungers and fullnesses *belong to them*, not anyone else. For instance, I may focus all my father-hunger thoughts and emotions on my father or stepfather. But the *hunger* isn't his; it's mine. And I have choices and decisions about how to address the relational hunger and/or fullness I associate with another person or experience. That includes choices and decisions that do and/or don't include that other person or experience.

Exploring Edges and Patterns

Edges are naturally challenging, uniquely personal, and happening right now. They are also where we learn Intuitive Eating by putting mindfulness into action. When exploring edges, only you and your body can speak to what is too much, just right, or too little. Reaching the edge isn't the journey's end; it's a place to explore and navigate. The rest of our life (and recovery) will have edges, so learning this practice can help us with every other edge we ever encounter.

In the end, it doesn't matter how often a yoga therapist, psychotherapist, dietitian, or other provider tells you about edges in general or your specific edge in this moment. You must be a willing participant in order to know *your* edge. The information is in your body, where you live. You can't find the information outside your body. You have to invite yourself to this party.

Exploring and testing edges can create confusion and/or floods of sensation and emotion. That's only natural when working through the tough practice of choosing the eating disorder or choosing the authentic self. The challenge is to expect edginess and uncertainty while trusting that the process leads to growth. In his 1997 advice to fellow artists, David Bowie captures the experience:

> If you feel safe in the areas you're working in, you're not working in the right area. Always go a little further into the water than you feel you're capable of being in. Go a little bit out of your depth. And when you don't feel like your feet are quite touching the bottom, you're just about in the right place to do something exciting.
>
> (Bowie, 1997)

Practicing discernment can reduce unconscious, confused, and/or fearful reactions to our edges. It gives us the power to pause, observe, and clarify our emotional, relational, and body edges; and then prepare to manage them.

There are not "right and wrong" answers in intuition, or Intuitive Eating. After years with black-and-white eating disorder thinking, that's hard for many clients to imagine. As cultural anthropologist Dr. Jennifer James writes: "Intuition is a combination of insight and imagination … without the direct intervention of reasoning. Once you can imagine something you can begin the process of creating it."

When one of my patients went on her senior class trip, she was scared of what might happen and how she'd respond. She didn't like going a week without talking to her therapist or me. Her therapist and I assured her that she'd done enough recovery work to navigate the situations she's likely to face. Returning to the rookie driver metaphor, I communicated my trust that she can like the idea of traveling to new places and enjoying the experiences. And I invited her to imagine that her experiences won't be "totaled" by getting lost, having a fender bender, or driving over a curb.

Metaphors, stories, and imagery are powerful recovery tools because they engage the client's imagination. For instance, we might ask a client to imagine their Intuitive Eating day as a canoe.

Canoes are light, agile vessels. They glide smoothly over the water with minimal sound, so you can hear nature. They are portable and portageable (carry them from one lake or river to the next along your journey). Canoes are easy to paddle and steer.

On the flip side (pun intended), canoes are easy to turn over, especially if the load is unevenly distributed. When a canoe is too front- or back-loaded, it's difficult to propel or steer. When a canoe is empty, it drifts away with the whims of wind and current, until a rock or branch snags it (and, perhaps, pokes a hole in the hull, and it sinks).

When a food log shows some morning and afternoon restriction, followed by evening overeating, we can visualize that *eating* day as a back-loaded or aft-heavy canoe. When a log shows over-full morning emotions, followed by calmer moods, we can visualize that *emotional* day as a front-loaded or bow-heavy canoe. Table 7.3 shows an example.

With or without metaphors, naming facilitates discernment of and conversations about patterns.

REGISTERED DIETITIAN (RD): I'm noticing that your eating days seem back-loaded this past week. It looks to me like you're eating very little until the evening, when there's calorie clustering. Do you see that pattern, or something else?

CLIENT: Yeah, you know, that is true. That's a pattern that I get into when I don't feel my hunger cues.

RD: That makes sense. What do you know about the times when it's hard to pick up your hunger cues?

CLIENT: Let's see. When I'm stressed, for sure.

RD: OK. Let's look at your log again. What pattern or patterns do you see in last week's emotional hunger/fullness column?

CLIENT: The numbers look pretty high from the morning until I get home from work. Then they drop.

RD: OK. Can you discern where you were feeling that pattern or that shift in your body?

CLIENT: Well, before work and at work, I was in my head the whole time. When I'm like that or I'm anxious, my jaw and my shoulders get tense.

RD: Can you discern where in your body you were feeling the shift when you got home?

CLIENT: That's hard. That's not so clear.

RD: Anything else you sensed or remember?

Table 7.3 Human Relationship Fullness

Event Time	Event	Who I Ate With/Where I Ate	Movement/Activity/Exercise	Pre-EIE Intention	Food Consumed	Physical Hunger/Fullness (Before/After)	Emotional Hunger/Fullness	Pacing: Fast (F) Moderate (M) Slow (S)	Symptoms	What I Noticed	What's Next Intention	Action Plan
7:30 am	Wake		Walk to subway. Took stairs vs. escalator							Woke up stressed and running late	To not let stress influence my eating	Eat breakfast ASAP
08:30	Breakfast	In office meeting with clients		Eat enough	½ muffin, coffee	4/5	8/8	M/S	Restrict	I can't feel my hunger. In fact, I feel so full of feelings I don't know if I'm hungry at all	To not let stress influence my eating	Eat morning snack at 11:00
11:30	Snack	At desk, alone		Eat regardless of mood/motivation	Vanilla yogurt, pack of trail mix	3/7	8/7	F	Eating fast	I felt anxious, stressed, irritable. I ate fast, did not really taste the food but did notice after I ate it all that I enjoyed the combination of flavors	To not let stress influence my eating	Eat lunch at 1:30. Ask co-worker to join

| 01:30 pm | Lunch | With Antonio at cafe | Walked to cafe and back to office. About 15 minutes each way | Take a break, connect with people | Ham and cheese on rye, pickle and chips (did not finish all; ate 2/3) | 5/9 | 7/6 | S | Restricted | I feel nauseous. I'm very full very fast and pushing myself to finish this meal. I noticed I was talking fast to Antonio but eating slow. I did notice the saltiness of the pickle. It reminded me of a Jewish deli where I grew up | To not let stress influence my eating | Mini-meal is next at 4:30. I already have it in my fridge at work |
| 04:30 | Mini-meal | In a meeting with my boss | | Eat for energy | Skipped— ugh! | 4 | 9 | NA | Skipped MM | My mini meal was ready to go and then my boss called me into his office. He's very critical of the project I'm working on for weeks. | Nourish my body now! | Get snack in before leaving office |

(Continued)

Table 7.3 (Cont.)

Event Time	Event	Who I Ate With/ Where I Ate	Movement/ Activity/ Exercise	Pre-EE Intention	Food Consumed	Physical Hunger/ Fullness (Before/ After)	Emotional Hunger/ Fullness	Pacing: Fast (F) Moderate (M) Slow (S)	Symptoms	What I Noticed	What's Next Intention	Action Plan
										I'm ready to scream. I feel angry. I have no appetite		
05:30	Snack	On the street on my way home by myself	Walked to subway	Making up for lost nutrients	Clif Bar, banana	3/4	8/7	F	None!	Feel hungry all of the sudden. After I ate my snack I still was a bit hungry. Now I have a craving for chips!	Do not go into the bodega for chips	Took another route home to bypass the place where they sell those BBQ chips I love
06:30	Waiting for dinner	Alone	10 push-ups, 50 sit-ups, 25 squats, 15	Tolerate feeling antsy		1	4			All of the sudden I'm starving I realized I'm	Eat dinner at moderate pace	Remind myself to check in, breathe,

Time	Meal	Setting	Plan	Food	Rating	Rating		Trigger	Thoughts/feelings	Coping	Action
		minutes of arm weights							pretty drained from all the stress today. Squeezed in 30 minutes of calisthetics hoping it would help me feel less stressed		and set an intention for moderate-paced meal
07:30	Dinner	With spouse, watching TV	Eat mindfully, moderate pacing	3 slices of pizza, salad with dressing	0/8	4/2	M	Overeat	I can tell I'm less stressed. I noticed how hard I tried to focus on even pacing. But I'm a bit over full and feel like I ate too much	Sit with feelings of fullness	Distract; watch my favorite show
09:30	Snack	With spouse, watching TV	Try to eat balanced snack	Apple and 2 Tbs peanut butter	4/8	2/1	F	Eating fast	Even though I wasn't very hungry I still wanted to eat. I love the smooth creamy peanut butter with crisp apple	Get to bed	Put on PJs

(Continued)

Table 7.3 (Cont.)

Event Time	Event	Who I Ate With/ Where I Ate	Movement/ Activity/ Exercise	Pre-EE Intention	Food Consumed	Physical Hunger/ Fullness (Before/ After)	Emotional Hunger/ Fullness	Pacing: Fast (F) Moderate (M) Slow (S)	Symptoms	What I Noticed	What's Next Intention	Action Plan
09:55	Snack	Standing up in my kitchen		None	2 servings of ice cream	8/9	1/0	M	Compulsive Eating	Feeling pretty numbed out	Get to bed	Washed face
10:30	Snack	On my phone, surfing the web		None	The rest of the pint of ice cream	9/10	0/0	S	Compulsive Eating	Ditto	Get to bed	Stop eating now and brush teeth

CLIENT: Well, now that I think about it, I remember wanting to numb out on Thursday night. That's the night I had pizza, ice cream, and binge-watched *Game of Thrones*.

RD: Is it fair to say that your emotional day was a front-loaded canoe?

CLIENT: Yeah. And I know what you're gonna say next. That's there a relationship between feeling emotionally overloaded and under-eating. Then, when I got home from work, I overate to numb and distract myself.

RD: What pattern or patterns do you see?

CLIENT: High emotion and low eating followed by overeating, numbed emotions, and still hungry.

RD: You nailed it. Here's my suggestion. Let's meal plan for the next three days, so you don't have back-loaded eating days. Then, use your food log and your journal to notice whether that affects the pattern or flow of your energy, anxiety, concentration, etc. on those days. When you meet with your therapist on Tuesday, and me next week, we highlight and look together at any patterns we recognize.

CLIENT: Worth a try, I suppose!

RD: Yeah. I find that this can really help people put their minds around what's happening. You may even end up with some knowledge—or wisdom—you can share with your therapist and/or me next time.

These conversations may seem labored or overly basic. But we tend to do this much unpacking early in Intuitive Eating. Once the person gets it, it's not confusing; they know the pattern. This knowledge opens the door to the intuitive practice of deciding what to do next.

Our clients will still experience times when they're flooded with feelings or feel emotionally starved. They want the pain to stop. The most familiar "make it stop" pattern revolves around eating disorder symptom use. At least twice a week, a client says:

> Oh great! Thanks a lot! My emotions are just too much to handle right now *and* you've gotten me to this "food can't fix that" part. OK, Intuitive Eating expert, I need to know what to do next! What's my substitute?

It's usually a letdown when I say:

> Well, there is no substitute. The main "antidote" is to sit with your feelings and let them inform you of what is happening emotionally. Bring that information to the emotional work you're doing with your treatment team. Share that information with a friend, and practice accepting their support and comfort. And, one more bit of information from all my years of this work: your bad days in Intuitive Eating are very important days.

In these moments of intense emotions, recovery-oriented distraction techniques can calm the brain so clients get clearer signals and can act intuitively. They *don't* deny or fix the problem and they don't substitute for recovery work. They are next things to do. Here are some examples.

- Riding the wave: when you have an urge to use symptoms, use a device that tells time and has an alarm. Then:
    a. Note the current time, notice the urge, and rate its intensity.
    b. Choose a distraction.
    c. Choose a length of time to engage in the distraction.
    d. Set the alarm or timer for that length of time.
    e. Engage in the distraction until the alarm rings: At 4:00 pm my urge rating is at a 10. I choose to distract by showering for 15 minutes and set the alarm for 4:15. When the alarm goes off, I revisit my urge and re-rate its intensity.If it's still high, I "ride the wave" again. If it's lower, I might move on to another activity (including other distraction techniques).

- Journaling: open up a page and start writing for five minutes. Go longer if you want or need to. If that seems out of reach, write about one of these topics: gratitude, breathing, a favorite movie, a friend, or your favorite smell.
- Play a board game: playing checkers, Monopoly, Boggle, etc. funnels energy into an engaging activity that's not over-stimulating (or life-and-death). Plus, you do it with other people! When other humans are not available you can solve crossword or sudoku puzzles; but do them on paper, so you avoid the seductive numbing of electronic games!
- Knitting: your hand/eye dexterity creates engaging but not over-stimulating (or life-and-death) patterns. You are awake, aware, creative and giving your hamster-brain a knit-tastic rest.
- Pets: playing with and petting pets are amazing distractions. Most of the time, pets willingly let you lean on them for comfort, compassion, and play. Walking a pet gets you from standing in front of the fridge to being outside. Petting your pet provides sensory comfort and refocuses attention to something fun and satisfying.
- Read a book: we agree with Ringo Starr in the *A Hard Day's Night* movie: "Books? I like books."

The people in our care have accomplished and learned a lot by the time they move into Intuitive Eating. However, that doesn't remove risk; we're actually upping the ante. We're inviting "failure." We ask clients to risk as-yet-unknown body experiences. We help them discern evidence that they will be safe if, for example, they deviate from a familiar protein source (like chicken) to an "as-yet-unknown" protein source (like yak). They practice trusting themselves (and their body's inner wisdom) to take the risk.

The evidence conveniently lies in their own body:

- My fullness/hunger cues will tell me when to start and stop eating.
- My body will recognize protein in the yak, even though I've never eaten yak.
- If I feel like I'm going to binge, my gut can say don't take three appetizers; two is safer.
- If I feel like I'm going to restrict, my gut can say don't take one appetizer; three is wiser.
- This appetizer was really good; I'd like to try it again.
- If I eat a little bit too little or a little bit too much, I will be OK.
- If I pause to check my physical and emotional hunger/fullness levels, I can know what to do next.

As Intuitive Eating progresses, between-session check-ins decrease for many patients. In sessions, the focus shifts to exploring, rather than constructing meal plans or planning shopping strategies. Their intensive and important recovery work is interpreting their life patterns. With continued practice, they refine their ability to identify issues, problems, and progress.

For example, a patient recently started our session by saying:

> You know, Maria, I remember us talking about the transition from work to home. I'm noticing that I have a really good handle on most things during the day, but there is still this thing that happens at night. I see an overeating pattern. I also recognize that I'm not overeating in the same compulsive ways I used to. But I do feel like I'm numbing out a little bit.

Not only did she discern the change in the intensity of her overeating, her tone and affect were calm while she described the situation. I saw this as evidence of discernment reducing reactivity while increasing perspective. She could present the issue calmly because she's well practiced in so many recovery skills. There's less fact-finding and more "what do we do next?" When I shared this observation, she responded: "Yeah. I'm already doing so many things right, so it's not such a big deal any more to identify a problem and then troubleshoot it with you."

Intuitive Eating also opens up our patients to excitement. One of my colleague's patients entered a session and enthusiastically announced:

> I went out with Sharee for dinner last night and feel proud that I knew what and how much to order without any stress. I just felt thrilled to be

there without my eating disorder in tow, because I've already done this eating thing a million times before. We talked and laughed the whole time. It was just great.

In our experience, the Intuitive Eating phase has a reliable arc. In the beginning it's rocky. We still rely on the skills and qualities of mindfulness, working on questions like: "What did you notice about your energy levels?"

As the arc continues, people get closer to intuiting their inner wisdom. We hear the language shift to "I really listened to myself and what I wanted next." and "I really enjoyed my food. I felt a lot more comfortable. I can't believe I said food and enjoy in the same sentence!"

"Calling Inner Wisdom: Come in Please!"

Remember when we said that mindfulness practice is not instant bliss? The same is true of inner wisdom practices. Let's take meditation or prayer for an example.

Prayer and meditation can sweep away mental and emotional debris, clearing space to develop pathways to inner wisdom. Simple enough to fit in a single sentence, right? Not so fast; literally.

Even experienced practitioners know that an hour of silent meditation or prayer often contains only five minutes of "quiet" mind or communion with God. Those "mastery moments" are powerful—and they pass. On the recovery journey, spiritual practices are essential. They also do more than plow wreckage to the side of the road.

Spiritual practices strengthen our inner dialogue around hope, trusting one's self, compassion, confidence, community, letting go, having faith, and being of service. They reveal our motivations and inform our intentions. Spiritual practices draw us closer to the truth within us, so we put that truth into action.

Well, at least it's simple enough to fit into three sentences, right? Yes and no. Spiritual practice is simultaneously simple, complex, obvious, opaque, frustrating, comforting. Like life itself, it's chock full of paradox. We never get *the* truth, the *whole* truth, and *nothing but* the truth. At the same time, we must practice rigorous honesty—and aim for *progress*, not perfection.

The practice draws us closer to truth. Paradoxically, drawing closer is more liberating and interesting than arriving at or capturing *the* truth (whatever that might look like). We see the ways that truth is simultaneously fixed and fluid.

In stillness, we can intuitively assemble our mindfulness "data" in order to create stronger and more developed connections with inner wisdom. The stillness serves us whether it feels serene, scary, comforting, uncomfortable, uncertain, and/or challenging. That's why it takes practice to sit with stillness. Remember, "when you don't feel like your feet are quite touching the bottom, you're just about in the right place to do something exciting."

During yoga therapy with my clients, we use guided meditations.

- Close your eyes and take a few deep, relaxing breaths.
- Imagine going up a ladder from your heart to a cloud.
- Then, imagine the cloud takes you on a journey to your favorite landscape; one that makes you feel safe.
- *(After a few moments)* Let the experience unfold.
- *(After a few moments)* Tell me what you notice. (Intuition is forming and informing the imagery.)
- Now, notice a door in your landscape. Tell us more about the door.
- Tell us what you notice about yourself while you experience the door.
- If you choose to open the door, let your experience unfold and describe what you notice. *(If the client chooses not to enter the door, we explore through other techniques.)*
- Notice a symbol or object that was left here as a gift for you.
- Let your experience unfold. Tell us what you are noticing about it. Tell us what you are noticing about yourself.
- Take your gift back through the door and to your landscape.
- Carry the gift with you on to the cloud.
- Bring it back down the ladder to your body.
- Keep your eyes closed as you settle back into your body. Sit up and take a few breaths.
- Consider this "gift" you've taken back with you. What would it be like to find meaning or a message through this symbol?
- What is this gift/symbol/object trying to communicate to you?
- How can you take its wisdom into your everyday life?
- Can you imagine a specific action you can take, guided by this wisdom?
- What would it be like to bestow gratitude on yourself for providing this experience and wisdom?

Choices and Decisions

During the practice of discernment, we come to recognize differentiation between people, places, and things. Differentiation reveals choices. Choices demand decisions. Decisions lead to action. Even inaction is action; as the old saying goes: "Not to decide is to decide."

Intuitive Eating leads clients toward self-accountability and responsibility. They make this progress by practicing—and experimenting with—choice, decision, and action.

- In this moment, I have to *choose* among options of what to do next:

  - Eat tuna or corned beef.
  - Purge or meditate or walk the cat or play checkers with my roommate.
  - Binge to numb my frustration or call my best friend to vent or walk the cat or play checkers with my roommate.

- In this moment, I have to *decide* what to do next:

  - Eat the tuna.
  - Walk the cat.
  - Binge to numb my frustration.
  - Nothing.

- In this moment, I have to do the next *action*:

  - Pick up the tuna and put it in my mouth.
  - Put a leash on the cat and walk out the door.
  - Get the package of cookies out of the cupboard and eat them.
  - Nothing.

After this choice, decision, and action cycle, we guide clients to ask challenging and necessary recovery questions:

- During each part of the cycle, what did I notice about my body, my brain, my emotions, my relationships, etc.?
- What is my relationship to choice and choosing?
- What is my relationship to deciding what to choose?
- What is my experience when deciding (remember that not to decide is to decide)?
- What did I learn about the action?
- What did I learn from taking the action?
- How does this inform my next go-round?

Of course, clients need to practice the distinct elements of the choice, decision, and action during non-eating hours, too. They improve access to their inner wisdom though exercising the muscles of choosing, deciding, acting, reflecting, learning, and using what they learn to inform the next round of life moments.

During Intuitive Eating, we explore the patient's entire day. We practice discerning and naming relationships, emotions, thoughts, etc. *in the moment* and through the lens of eating patterns.

We guide people in our care to practice curiosity in every choice in their unique life. "What am I noticing about my experience in this moment? What am I noticing about my fullness/hunger patterns? How do they relate to me and what I decide to do next?"

We invite them to explore these questions when:

- I have a fight with my girlfriend.
- I'm awed by the Grand Canyon.
- My boss does this, that, and the other thing.
- I have a loving connection.
- I spend one-on-one time with my friend.
- I feel excited.
- I have a spiritual experience.
- I am creative.
- I spend time with a group of friends.
- I'm over the line of my edge.
- I am bored.
- I'm feeling anger.
- I feel empathy.
- I feel impatient.
- I feel empty.
- I feel full.
- I feel satisfied.
- My body is sick.

With consistent practice, our patients gain deeper understanding of their patterns of discerning, choosing, deciding, and acting. They intuit how to approach the next moments, days, months, and years. As Frances G. Wickes wrote in *The Inner World of Childhood*: "Without intuition there would be no vision of future possibilities."

Every repetition of recovery discerning, choosing, deciding, and acting strengthens healing by deepening new neural pathways. And every repetition weakens eating disorder discerning, choosing, deciding, and acting by pruning old neuropathways. Ultimately, clients learn to value themselves and their bodies enough to stop abusing themselves and their bodies.

An Intuitive Eating patient described going to a deli without planning her lunch beforehand.

> As soon as I went through the door, I smelled tuna fish. Without thinking, I said "Hey, that's what I want!" I went back a few days later for lunch, but the fish smell felt gross. The sauerkraut smelled great, though, so I got a Reuben. It's a little weird. What's going on?

Here's what's going on. For years, an entrenched eating disorder blocked her natural physiologic cravings. Now, the communication channels between brain, digestion, nutrition needs, organs, etc. are opening up. The sensation of smelling fish opens the channels that unconsciously discern a body need (perhaps for omega-3 fatty acids), which then opens a channel to *wanting* fish, not just *needing* it. This is radically different than impulsive or compulsive behavior. Without even planning or thinking ahead, she intuited an in-the-moment nutritional and emotional desire, and what to do next: order and eat a tuna salad sandwich on rye.

On the days when tuna smells fishy and sauerkraut smells fine, she might be intuiting her body's need for vitamin C, vitamin K, vitamin U, magnesium, and gut flora (sauerkraut) and/or its need for riboflavin, niacin, protein, iron—and omega-3 fatty acids (corned beef). Without even planning or thinking ahead, she intuited an in-the-moment nutritional and emotional desire, her choice, and her what-to-do-next decision: order and eat a Reuben on rye.

This woman's "old" neural pathways reinforced rigid "if-then" eating disorder thoughts and beliefs like:

- If fish (or sauerkraut) *ever* smells fishy to me, even once, then I can *never* eat it again.
- I read that tuna has mercury, so it'll kill me.
- I read that tuna has 5,000 calories, so I can't eat it.
- Sauerkraut is fermented, like compost, so I can't eat it.

At the deli, she is experiencing and using new neural pathways and neuroplasticity she developed during recovery. She can remember the old pathway while using its data to *inform* what she does next. Of course, she knows the old way—and can choose it. At the same time, she knows/intuits that neither the old way nor her memories of it *dictate* what she does next.

Naturally, new "what I do next" choices are risky and/or feel risky. So, during Intuitive Eating, people practice taking calculated risks. Informed choices and calculated risks ingrain new neural pathways that facilitate flexible "if-then" thoughts and beliefs like:

- I can test the hypothesis of my worst fear: "If I eat this sandwich, then I will gain 100 pounds by the morning." That's ridiculous; hypothesis invalidated.
- If tuna smells fishy today, then I can still crave it next week.
- If I order and eat a Reuben, cobb salad, or any of 25 other things in this deli, then I can fill some of my physiological needs.
- If my friend and I eat at the deli together, then I can fill some of my emotional and relational needs, and worry less about mercury in my tuna, the wilt on that piece of lettuce, or the deli's Yelp rating.

My client can practice trusting her inner eater and her inner wisdom in a deli and everywhere else in her life.

Food Fears and Food Preferences

Every professional working with eating disorders recognizes food fears, and how endemic they are in our patients. We address those fears (implicitly and explicitly) during therapy sessions, physician visits, meal plans, and more. For example, therapeutic meals in a treatment program are, in effect, food fear exposure therapy.

Effective eating disorders treatment invites open acknowledgment of food fears and makes them safe to discuss. Ideally, early in treatment, these approaches facilitate restorative eating that addresses patients' malnutrition.

Full disclosure: those conversations frequently include battles over the accurate definition of "preference" (liking one person, place, or thing better than another person, place, or thing). More precisely, we're battling over the eating disorder's definition of "preference" (shifting and distorting the meaning to reinforce denial and symptomatology). Some clients have difficulty disentangling "preference" from eating disorder thinking. This makes it hard to associate "preference" with choice, discernment, and intuition:

- "I prefer one-pound bags of chips over single-serving bags."
- "I never eat more than a half-ounce of soy for my protein."
- "I only like ice cream (*easy to purge*) and I hate peanut butter (*very hard to purge*)."

As treatment progresses, these approaches encourage food flexibility, like trying green beans. And, a few weeks later, trying asparagus. And, a few months later, trying bok choy. But the eating disorder continues its magical defining (a subspecialty of magical thinking):

- "I kept down that half-cup of egg salad, but mayonnaise is still abhorrent."
- "One cup of egg salad was fine, but I prefer two more cups, and a lot more mayonnaise."
- "I ate peanut butter for my evening snack, but it felt like concrete in my stomach. It's hard to get down and I had to keep it down, because purging it would hurt too much. Never again."

It's a huge step from the state of paralyzing food fear to tentative experiments in food flexibility. It's another huge step from tentative food flexibility to feeling safe with food flexibility. Still, the recovery path doesn't end here.

To fully recover, people in our care must make the next huge leap into knowing:

- what my unique body prefers to eat
- what I prefer to eat.

Recovery doesn't demand that all preferences are 100 percent in sync 100 percent of the time. But recovery does demand that they are known and/or intuited.

One strategy is creatively using the three words *within* preference: prefer, refer, and reference. This interpretation describes communication of "I prefer" suggestions between the body, mind, intuition, and self. I reference the body's encyclopedia of knowledge about what I prefer. I refer back to my body to discern what I prefer; e.g.: chocolate ice cream more than vanilla ice cream.

Prefer, refer, and reference are the polar opposites of an eating disorder's rigid, rule-driven, fear-based, so-called "preferences."

As clients begin moving into Mastered Eating, they know and/or intuit what they like to eat, what they don't like to eat, and what their bodies prefer. Their preferences almost always serve recovery, the body, and the self. Their eating and food preferences are balanced, fluid, and fixed.

Wait a minute! How and why can it be fluid *and* fixed? Because, over time, what we need and prefer change in some ways and remain fixed in other ways. Some people I know provide a good illustration:

- Twin, 40-something women who don't like mayonnaise. One of them never eats anything with mayonnaise, while the other occasionally eats tuna salad. They've never had an eating disorder, and their mayonnaise dislike isn't a product of pathological fear or rigidity. Rather, it appears to be inherited. Most of their paternal ancestors avoided mayonnaise because: "As Grandma Eleanor used to say, it feels slimy." While both women (and all of their ancestors) have quirks, it also appears coincidental that one of them married a spouse who doesn't eat *any* condiments.

- A 40-something man with anorexia who rigidly despised mayonnaise. Even its smell made him nauseous. Like many survivors of child sexual abuse, he associated creamy "semen-like" foods (mayo, yogurt, sour cream, etc.) with his trauma. Nearly a year of Structured Eating, intensive trauma therapy, and trauma-informed yoga practice passed before he tried a half-teaspoon of mayonnaise on a turkey sandwich. He eventually tolerated potato salad during Mindful Eating, when he wrote "disgusting texture" in his food logs, but also noted "tangy taste is nice." Continuing to experiment during Intuitive Eating, he noticed that "my tongue and throat seem to like the moisture and viscosity of mayo in food." The recovery process unblocked the channels sending "I prefer mayo" messages between his brain, mouth, throat, and gut. He learned: (1) his eating disorder and PTSD despised mayonnaise; and (2) in recovery, he likes foods that are made with blended oil, egg yolk, and vinegar or lemon juice. He doesn't like the associations it once evoked, and that's just fine.

The challenges are also complex when someone with an eating disorder fears and/or avoids an entire category of food.

I once had a client who was a dancer, avid vegetarian, and very motivated to recover from her eating disorders. When discussing her body's urgent weight restoration needs, I expressed concern that a vegetarian diet wouldn't contain all the needed macronutrients. She gave me many reasons why her yogic background and life values meant she could not abandon vegetarianism.

Sharing my own background and extensive training in yoga, I explained my yogic commitment to feeding my body what it needs. My yoga practice taught me that my body preferred getting its optimal protein from animal foodstuffs.

As we moved from structured to mindful to intuitive phases, my words about *my* body stuck with her. As a dancer and recovering anorexic, her body demanded adequate nutrients to get through each day. One day she told me that, despite her wish to remain vegetarian, she believed her body preferred animal protein. She also acknowledged a deep fear of giving up her vegetarian identity.

I invited her to look at this as an exploration. She didn't need to make a permanent commitment to meat and fish. She could listen to her body and how it responds to animal protein. She agreed to this and wandered through a process of slowly weaving meat and fish into her diet. Ultimately, she invited—and decided—that her body preferred animal protein. By referring to her body for what it needs and prefers, her animal protein preference felt like truth. For the time being, she made the decision to accept this and let go of her identity as a vegetarian.

That was also the time when we both knew she was transitioning into Mastered Eating.

Bibliography

Bowie, D. (1997). Life advice. interview. https://www.youtube.com/watch?v=7HqTQyQ6wc0

Desai, R., Tailor, A., and Bhatt, T. (2015). Effects of yoga on brain waves & structural activation: A review. *Complementary Therapies in Clinical Practice*, 21(2), 112–118.

James, J. *Thinking in the Future Tense: Leadership Skills for a New Age* (New York: Simon and Schuster, 1996).

Kelly, J. *Dads and Daughters: How to Inspire, Support and Understand Your Daughter* (New York: Broadway Books, 2002).

Maine, M. *Father Hunger: Fathers, Daughters and Food*, 2nd edition (Carlsbad, CA: Gurze Books, 2004).

Shinn, F.S. *The Game of Life and How to Play It* (New York: self-published, 1925. Reprinted, New York: Penguin Group, 2009).

Tribole, E. and Resch, E. *Intuitive Eating: A Revolutionary Program that Works* (New York: St. Martin's Press, 1995).

Wickes, F.G. *The Inner World of Childhood: A Study in Analytical Psychology*. (Boston: Sigo Press, 1988).

8 Mastered Eating

People are sometimes skeptical, confused, or leery when we talk about Mastered Eating. Doesn't that imply "perfect" eating? Isn't it sterile and rigid? If rigid pursuit of perfection is the problem in so many eating disorders, how can Mastered Eating be a solution, or something to strive toward?

Those are natural, reasonable questions. The answer lies in what we mean by mastery.

We all have the capacity to master skills, if we practice. At a young age, most of us master communicating through a language and reading in a language. If your body is ambulatory, you can master walking (after falling down a lot). Walking is complex; to take a single step, humans must integrate dozens of muscles and countless synapses. Yet athletes who run four-minute miles still trip over curbs. Walking is more than the sum of its parts: activated muscles, bones, and neural signals.

This phase of recovery and life calls us to master skills and relationships that are harder to define than walking, reading, and talking.

Let's think back to tennis master Serena Williams. Or, choose a master in some other field, like Yo-Yo Ma in classical music, Annie Leibovitz in photography, or Common in rap, writing, acting, and philanthropy.

I see some common characteristics in these masters and their work:

- They seem to have unusual focus and the ability to enter a "zone."
- Their focus, zone, and mastery never produce perfection.
- They have graceful relationships with their multiple skills and gifts.
- They are grateful for their teachers, their talents, and even their competitors.
- Words can't fully describe their mastery, or its evidence (e.g., the tone Ma's cello makes or the flow of Williams' game).
- The masters' own words can't fully describe their mastery.
- Their mastery seems to be more than the sum of its parts.
- They practice their art or craft with devotion, while knowing that practice can't guarantee mastery, flawlessness, or "success."

- Much of their mastery is mysterious, yet we sense a vibrant spirit radiating from it.
- Their mastery is awe-inspiring.

Nevertheless, we must accept the fact that this is a book, and thus we must use words to discuss mastery.

As they progress in Mastered Eating, clients frequently report "Eureka!" moments of inspiration, clarity, or intuition. These "mastery moments" happen when our brain generates short-burst, high-frequency gamma-waves, produced when whole neurons fire in sync. The highest-frequency brain waves are gamma-waves.

Because they're so fast, they can instantaneously process information from multiple other brain waves. Researchers are finding correlations between gamma-wave activity and self-control, natural joy, compassion, and increased sense awareness. Science continues to illuminate how and where intuition happens within the body.

By their very nature:

- Gamma-wave bursts can't be forced or scheduled for Thursday, the 13th at 3:00.
- Eating disorders smother a person's "Eureka!" capacity and their access to authentic inspiration, clarity, or intuition.
- Spiritual and yoga practices like meditation can facilitate Aha! moments of inspiration, clarity, or intuition.

Paradoxically, high-frequency gamma-waves are most likely to appear when a brain crosses the "threshold" between its slow-frequency alpha-waves and even slower theta-waves. Many everyday practices can "quiet" the mind and body, pause reactivity, and bring our brain waves closer to the alpha-theta threshold:

- meditation
- a hot shower (I get my best ideas in the shower!)
- dancing, singing, drumming, and other repetitive motion activities
- prayer or chanting
- yoga
- knitting.

Mastery moments aren't permanent, uninterrupted, or uninterruptible. Psychologist Mihaly Csikszentmihalyi suggests that mastery is a state of flow in which the person performs an activity with "energized focus," full involvement, and single-minded immersion. Mastery is more than the sum of our talents, competency, and proficiency. In mastery moments, we access previously inaccessible ways of knowing, sensing, and doing. Mastery transforms or transcends what we currently believe we can know, sense, and do.

Csikszentmihalyi says we get "in the zone" by holding the tension between skills we own, challenges we have, wisdom we receive, and as-yet-invisible potential. While emotions are contained and channeled, they are also positive, energized, and aligned with the task at hand (eating, rapping, or living, for example). This makes neuroscientific sense. Our nervous system can only process so much information in a given time period. When someone enters a super-focused state, stimuli outside the area of focus state (such as eating disorder thoughts) can't enter our brain.

In our experience, the sustained practice of acting on inner wisdom eventually provides the people in our care with mastery moments.

A Mastered Eating Story

A woman wakes up "in the mood" for eggs. She makes toast while scrambling two eggs. She smashes some avocado on to her toast and pours a glass of juice. She mutters: "that was delicious" as she puts her plate into the sink. She grabs another slice of avocado before jumping in the shower.

An unremarkable story, amazing story, or a complex story? All of these three, because this person is a mastered eater, fully recovered from an eating disorder. We may not see the complexity until we look under the nutritional hood and find:

- She wakes up in the morning and instinctively knows she's hungry.
- She doesn't need to consult a clock or meal plan because her circadian rhythm and internal signals are synched with mealtimes.
- Her body communicates its needs via an "I'm in the mood" message. She responds by organizing, making, and eating two eggs, toast, avocado, and juice.
- She doesn't wonder *if or how* she will get a chance to eat.
- The idea of skipping the meal never enters her mind (she's been eating breakfast every day for a very long time).
- She eats varied combinations of balanced breakfasts, so her body has nutritional imprints based on her specific needs.
- She's a bit hungry when done and trusts her body will figure it out.
- She is present for and responds to the meal's flavors.
- This breakfast was exactly what *she* wanted and what *her body* needed. Even amidst the hustle of the morning, she finds peace and gratitude for her body.
- She is now ready to move on with her day.

The story is amazing because it illustrates a person rising from the depths of eating disorders to masterfully integrate a synchronized body rhythm (including hunger and fullness cues), trust "in the mood for" cravings to communicate body needs, trust that the body will respond accordingly or signal if something is "wrong," troubleshooting, and grace.

At the same time, her eating mastery shifts the story to unremarkable. She is just doing her thing. Her actions are natural and carefree. She moves into, through, and beyond the experience with ease. And that is remarkable.

Foundations

People fully recovered from eating disorders are mastered eaters. Some people still journeying toward full recovery have mastered their eating. The "Mastered Eating" phase moves beyond eating with intuition and instinct alone. It integrates spirit, soul, spirituality, purpose, and other transcendent responses to life.

In yoga terms, treatment and recovery guide our clients to be living vessels of the central yoga tenets called *yamas* (restraints or avoidances) and *niyamas* (duties or observances).

Every treatment modality encourages clients to practice non-violence/non-self-harm, truthfulness, non-stealing, non-hoarding, and the right use of energy (the *yamas*). Every treatment modality encourages clients to practice a burning desire to change; acceptance; self-purification (e.g., clearing away eating disorder thoughts); self-study; and surrender (the *niyamas*). These principles and practices are at the heart of self-mastery and self-awakening. They call people to acceptance, caring, and purpose.

Perhaps paradoxically (or perhaps not), practicing *yamas* and *niyamas* elevates and widens our clients' perspective. In the crisis of active eating disorders, a person's view of reality continually narrows. It's as if the disorder leaves visible only five degrees of life's circle. During treatment and recovery, clients begin to see 20, 100, or 180 degrees of their life.

The self-mastered eater grows closer to 300 or more degrees of perspective on their eating, relationships, and life. They learn to look back with compassion and look forward with confidence.

They grow closer to embodying their true essence. In their recovery, they find the way to a safe, squatter-free home. They live less burdened by symptoms and less trapped by denial. They live with understanding that food, body, eating, situations, and days are not good or bad; wins or losses. They are filled with lessons, growth, and development of the soul experience. Here's a story a former client shared:

> I'm recovered from my eating disorder (ED) for a long time. But I recently connected some dots that surprised me. I was allowing ED "energy" into some of my relationships—one in particular. I felt that I was never enough for this person. I believed I never did enough or worked hard enough. I felt like I couldn't stay far enough in the background. Once I finally saw the ways I was repeating my ED patterns with a years-later personal relationship, I saw my part in a new way. And I stopped. I've ended the relationship for now, and

maybe for much longer. The whole situation got me thinking (for the first time) about the patterns in my relationship with one of my siblings when we were kids. *That* was like my ED relationship, too, years before I ever had an eating disorder.

Look, I do not believe that my childhood relationships caused my ED, or that my ED caused the relationship I just ended. That's not what this is about. It's like, for the first time, I realized that these past and present relationships had less to do with the other person than I thought. The way *I was* in those relationships was the way *I went* through the world.

I feel like I'm taking responsibility for my part—without blaming myself or feeling guilty about this (like I always did during the ED). Instead, this new picture of my old relationships with my sibling and my ED seems more well-lit and clearer. My part is better lit, too. I'm being an adult, and not continuing to react like a kid. So, I'm feeling much different about my sibling, their part, and their experience in our relationship.

All this seems to "light a way" to do my part differently. That means working to be more true to myself and to be more compassionate with others. I don't know what that means right now for me and my sibling (if anything). Right now, in this moment of clarity, I just feel sad for both of us and wish I could reach back and give us both big hugs. And that's way better than where I was before now.

It may sound weird to say but breaking off the recent relationship *surprised* me into breaking free from being handcuffed by outdated and distorted views of myself and relationships that matter to me.

Creating lasting recovery is not easy; it takes chemical, mental, emotional, spiritual, and physiological recalibration. Fortunately, we are all recovering from some past experiences, memories, feelings, and so on. As we locate lost parts of ourselves, we come to realize that we already have what we need to heal, to be present, to love, and so forth.

As Trappist monk Thomas Merton said: "We have what we seek. It is there all the time, and if we give it time, it will make itself known to us." Since humans are inherently imperfect, our seeking will inevitably reveal imperfection. Thus, mastery simultaneously and paradoxically seeks the ultimate and lets go of illusory perfection.

Mastery Skills

As we mentioned in the Introduction, people in treatment and recovery regularly ask: "Who am I without my eating disorder?" Early in recovery, the question may feel overwhelming. In seven words, the question captures:

- the enormous leap of faith clients must make
- the terror of stepping away from familiar eating disorder ways, and risking eating disorder retribution
- the terror of stepping away from familiar eating disorder ways and being overwhelmed by life
- the terror of stepping toward the as-yet-unknowable path of recovery.

By the time clients transition to Mastered Eating, their terror has eased. Mastered Eating calls them to ask deeper and wider questions, such as: "Who am I *beyond* my eating disorder?" Such pondering lies at the heart of a sacred yoga *niyama* (duty or obligation) known as *svadhyaya*.

Self-Study

Svadhyaya is the practice of self-study. It's not anything like studying (or cramming) for an exam. There is no test, GPA, or other numerical value. Life defies grading, report cards, or scorecards.

Svadhyaya includes looking for what was lost *and* looking for what is still hidden. Like the rest of yoga practice and philosophy, *svadhyaya* invites us to study without judgment of, expectations for, or attachment to what we find.

That's not easy to do. With our clients, we talk about self-study in practical terms. For example, there is no such thing as a bad day for studying the self-data they already know how to mindfully notice. For instance:

- Body changes can be signals to address something new or old in my life.
- Revisiting eating disorder patterns can shed new light on the past and the present.
- Symptoms (from an eating disorder or anything else) are important messengers that there is something of imbalance in my self.
- Lapse or relapse can inform me that I am in a new layer of life and self.

I sometimes invite patients to envision Mastered Eating like a video game, where "mastering" one level means breaking into a whole new level of challenges. The new level has more bells and whistles, but the player is stronger and has more weapons to face as-yet-unknown possibilities. *Svadhyaya* lets them know when they've broken through to the next level.

Svadhyaya also lets patients know when they're reaching (or hurtling through) walls or ceilings into levels they've never seen; and thus don't (yet) have enough tools—or the right tools—to cope with the experience.

All of us face stressful life situations, like the death of a loved one. We're affected by shock and grief, no matter how far along the balanced-living path we've traveled. Loss and other stress may or may not lead to lapses or relapses for people recovered or recovering from eating disorders. If lapses or relapses do occur, we guide clients back to recovery practices, and suggest that their familiarity with those practices is a huge asset.

We have a patient whose eating was on cruise control after working very hard in recovery. Recently, their husband died. The client began binge eating after years of not using any symptoms. Embarrassed and confused, they re-entered treatment.

THEM: I'm so ashamed of myself for being back at square one.

REGISTERED DIETITIAN (RD): There is no such thing as square one for you. You have learned so much about yourself, your body, your eating, and your life.

THEM: That's why I can't believe I let this happen.

RD: Sometimes we don't have skills to respond to an experience because the experience never occurred in our lives before. This new situation may require a screwdriver when you only have a hammer and saw. Or it may require a flat-head screwdriver, and you only have a Phillips head. You never needed "I lost a spouse" tools before.

THEM: I understand that, but it feels like a I'm a failure. My recovery is so important to me.

RD: Do your grief, stress, and the amount of upheaval seem like they are beyond your capacity to cope right now?

THEM: Absolutely.

RD: Is it possible that your eating disorder symptoms rushed in to numb the feelings? After all, it's a familiar coping mechanism that worked in the past when you felt overwhelmed.

THEM: Yes, but I still can't believe I let my eating disorder back in. This is a disaster.

RD: I don't believe this lapse will define you. You have years of experience recovering from your eating disorder and living without your symptoms. You already know that you'll work hard to manage your symptoms.

THEM: I don't know if I can. Life is too much right now and bingeing is soothing my pain.

RD: I know.

THEM: I'm scared this is going to take over again. That I won't be able to stop looking to the eating disorder and the symptoms as my security blanket.

RD: I hear you. Let me ask you this: is it possible that your symptoms are informing you in any way?

THEM: Well, yeah. They're showing me how desperate and miserable I feel about Tony dying.

RD: Let me ask you this: is it possible that the bingeing is challenging or prodding you to find new resources, skills, people to help walk with your grief?

THEM: I guess it's possible, in theory. And I believe that you believe it's possible.

RD: I believe that might be what's happening. Are you willing to work on this theory with your therapist? And to work on this theory with me in our yoga and nutrition sessions?

THEM: I suppose. But I'm not sure that will help me. I'm still scared about what's gonna happen next and how I can live without Tony.

RD: I believe it will help you. And *you* will help you, because you're not at square one. I've known you for a long time. You already know about recovery. You've trusted the process when it wasn't linear, and you couldn't clearly see how it would turn out. This is not your first rodeo. I've got your back. *Your body has your back.* Let's get to work.

After a few months of weekly sessions with their therapist and dietitian, we saw movement:

RD: How was your week?

THEM: OK. I've been able to eat on schedule better and have a bit more flexibility. I only had a few compulsive eating episodes this week.

RD: What kind of information did your symptoms provide you with?

THEM: At night, when I'm in pain and grieving in bed, I want to eat. I know it won't really help. Sometimes I listen to a guided meditation and go to sleep. Sometimes I just cry and pray I'll be OK. Sometimes I binge.

RD: This sounds huge for you.

THEM: How? I'm still bingeing to cope.

RD: Yes, *and* you adopted other coping mechanisms.

THEM: Yes. I feel I'll be able to move past these symptoms because I see their role but I also know I don't need them. I need to grieve sometimes. I'm trying to be patient and compassionate.

RD: I've got your back. *Your body has your back.* Let's continue to work.

After a few more months of less-frequent sessions with their therapist and dietitian, we glimpsed signs of mastery:

THEM: I went another week without symptoms!

RD: Amazing! Tell me more!

THEM: It felt like Bill Murray in *Groundhog Day* every few days. I would get to a point in the day or the week where I would use symptoms. But I could tell they were no longer serving me.

RD: How could you tell?

THEM: Well, I have something to compare them to. I'm starting to feel safe grieving with my family and friends and my treatment team. My eating disorder is not a teammate.

RD: You seem excited and relieved.

THEM: Yeah, I think I am. So, one night, I just said "no more." I got through one week and then another week. I want to get through more. I accept that I might have an episode here and there but, like you said, it will not define me.

RD: I could not be prouder of you, your bravery, your willingness to understand that you are healing, and your recovery can be a part of that.

THEM: I actually feel motivated. Like I want to do this for me, my family, and Tony. He would not want me to suffer with symptoms.

RD: Good for you.

THEM: I think I can go a month between sessions. I'll call you if I need you.

RD: You know I have your back. Your body and spirit are proving they have your back. I'll see you in a month, unless you need to come in sooner.

Both clinician and client must self-study how we respond to lapses and relapses. Clinicians must practice welcoming and accepting these clients, and not shame or judge them (even inadvertently).

We say the following to our clients, and encourage them to say this to themselves:

> Trust your discomfort—it has data for you. It's part of your inner wisdom. Your inner wisdom/soul says: Let me into your decision making. Let the gut feeling I share be a guide. Let me help to reveal the reason(s) you don't feel comfortable with this situation. Trust in me and listen to what feels right. I've got your back.

Self-Mentoring

In recovery, yoga therapy, and virtually every other growth or healing tradition, practitioners rely on mentors. For example, every monk has a spiritual director with whom they examine and explore what the monk "hears" in prayer and meditation.

As in other traditions, recovery and yoga call us to practice *self-mentoring*. Indeed, practice itself is a self-mentoring process familiar to most experienced psychotherapists, dietitians, physicians, electricians, heavy equipment operators, chefs, schoolteachers, and so on.

A yoga therapy mentor has always supervised my work with clients, my technique, and the inner work I must do. When I started providing yoga therapy, my *self*-mentoring was much more critical than my mentor's mentoring was. Fortunately, after years of practice, I learned to master authentic self-mentoring in real time. I'm not perfect, but I can be embodied in my self while simultaneously being fully present to my client. In each moment, I can dialogue with myself without judgment. While working with a client, I can ask myself:

- What was my intention in saying "good"?
- Can I consider how to create a smoother transition?
- I see my agenda was here in the room when I asked this question.
- I notice I want her to get something out of this session. Do I do this technique and risk it?

With time, my self-mentoring inner dialogue became energy, like an internal wind I experience flowing one way or turning another way. Each time I consider and clarify intentions, expectations, and agenda, I create a clearer channel for my client to receive their session.

One of our greatest thrills in this work is witnessing clients self-mentor. I have a 50-something patient with a trauma history, who is recovering from bulimia. She's had a complicated relationship with exercise. Like many patients, she used it to burn calories and get "in shape." Other times, she had no motivation to move for fear exercise would stir trauma memories.

During treatment, she embraced yoga and did some amazing work in our yoga therapy group. Now a year or so out of treatment, her eating disorder support sessions are less frequent and prescriptive. She recently joined a local gym where her recovery-focused practice is to exercise based on how she feels. She explained:

> I'm not looking for my personal best time anymore. I'm exercising to honor my boundaries. If that means walking instead of running, that's OK. I have to work at it, though. Last week, after a really long day, my judgey voice started pressuring me to go to the gym. I had to stop and think—or notice—before I realized how tired I was. I honored that and decided that taking the evening off was the right thing to do.

She wanted to know why I had such a big smile on my face. I replied:

> I just started thinking about exercising to achieve a "personal best" time. Now, you're moving with awareness, exercising within your energy, and resting when you need to. That sounds like using exercise to get a best *personal* time.

She got the wordplay and laughed. We both acknowledged her major leap of mastering gym time to serve her relationship with her body and self. In the process of showing what is and what can be, mastery debunks old stories of how and what things used to be.

Self-mentoring is an endless path to deeper knowledge, acceptance, gratitude, and joy. My fellow dietitian and yoga teacher Lisa Diers expressed this recently while reflecting on leaving an eating disorders treatment agency where she worked for many years.

Today marks exactly *two years* since I said goodbye to people and familiarity that I held so dear to my heart. Although I had a deep knowing that all would be OK. I worked hard to remember that sensation when in the midst of *challenging change*. Those are the moments to *rise up, meet it, greet it,* and *welcome* the lessons that *transformation* will bring. *Thank you!* I could not have made this transition without all the amazing family, friends, colleagues, and people in my life!

Earlier in recovery, moving into unknown levels of life while feeling joy seems impossible to the people in our care. Mastery shows that it's doable.

Surrendering to Care

Care is central to recovery. Clients are people in our care. We give them our care and care about them. Depending on the situation, we challenge and/or invite them to receive care from others. When a person agrees to enter treatment and/or to be a part of recovery, they experience care, whether or not they believe they are worthy of care.

Dietitians frequently hear eating disorders reject authentic care in statements like: "If you really cared about me, you would/wouldn't make me eat that!" The client (or their eating disorder) is convinced that "making" them eat/not eat is cruel, arbitrary, controlling, and disrespectful. Nonetheless, clinicians know that it is real care.

Some clients never cared for themselves before, while others have lost track of how to do it. In recovery, clients practice caring for the body, instead of practicing the eating disorder's cunning pseudo-care. They self-care by:

- eating to nourish their body
- mindfully noticing thoughts and feelings
- discerning how they correspond, respond, and react to their symptom patterns
- listening hard to gut instincts and trusting intuition to accompany them through fear
- nourishing their soul and their communities.

We introduce this last point by discussing the last *niyama: ishvarapranidhana*. *Pranidhana* means dedication, devotion, and self-surrender. *Ishvara* means the "source" to which/whom we dedicate, devote, and surrender our self.

Ishvarapranidhana "surrender" doesn't mean stopping all effort, resigning from life, or waving a white flag. Instead, *ishvarapranidhana* invites the "surrender" of turning over our will and our life to the *care* of a supreme life Source, God, universal consciousness, Creator, Great Spirit, gods, or other power(s) greater than ourselves. We find this concept of "turning over" surrender in many spiritual and religious devotions:

- I give You myself—my body, my mind, and my heart—to do with as You best see fit.
- O Allah! Thee do we serve.
- Thy will, not mine, be done.
- Lead me from death to life, from falsehood to truth. Lead me from despair to hope, from fear to trust. Lead me from hate to love, from war to peace.
- Creator, you know what will be beautiful in what we do. Give me how to live my life well.
- Let go, let God.

Surrendering seems antithetical to our culture's self-sufficient, you're-on-your-own values. Surrendering to an eating disorder can seem self-destructive. Many clients find surrender concepts more accessible when we discuss "letting go" as the process of *ending*, *transitioning*, and *beginning*, not resignation.

Imagine being a proud parent removing training wheels from your child's bicycle. They have the skills to pedal, steer, and balance the bike with *four* wheels. Keeping the training wheels on will stall their riding potential. You know they are ready for the next risky and necessary step.

Your child is excited, a little afraid, confident, and ready. They hope they don't fall, but you (and some part of them) know that falling teaches the final skills of riding on *two* wheels. You're still present as they wobble down the sidewalk the first few times. But they and their bike no longer need you in the same way. You both know that bike will take your child to all sorts of places without you.

Nevertheless, you look on with pride (and a little fear), while they awkwardly try to control each distinct element of biking. They look down to monitor a foot on the pedal, which throws their body off balance, and the bike tips over. They keep getting back on, even when they get frustrated or need a Band-Aid. They learn important patterns. "If I lean too far over, I will fall." They're no longer scared but exhilarated. They want to get this. As your voice grows more distant, their inner voice gets louder: "I got this!" They still wobble for a while, but they're eager to practice this new way of being and moving.

Suddenly your child integrates the distinct elements, without either of you quite knowing how they did it. They do that awe-inspiring thing we call letting go. They right the bike and keep their balance. In no time, they masterfully navigate the ins and outs of the neighborhood. Without training wheels, they experience freedom, scenery, the wind, and the neighbors while they ride. They may sing or take a deep breath in awe, knowing: "I got wheels, I know how to ride them, I'm going places I've never been before."

We can find freedom at any age through surrender or letting go of "old" stories and perceptions. My co-author Joe's favorite saying (attributed to Mark Twain, Ann Landers, and probably others) speaks to this:

> When I was in my 20s, all I cared about was what other people thought of me. When I reached my 40s, I decided not to give a damn what anyone thought of me. When I reached my 60s, I realized that people weren't ever thinking about me in the first place.

It's human nature to expend mental and emotional energy worrying about what others think of us, even though:

• They're naturally engaged with thinking about themselves.
• Their opinion of us (if any) is more about them than it is about us (plus, it's beyond our control).

Ironic? Paradoxical? Laughable? No. It's all three. So is human nature.

That's why psychotherapy, *ishvarapranidhana*, spiritual practice, recovery—and parts of our human nature—guide us to practice acceptance, gratitude, compassion, fidelity, patience, intention, dedication, devotion, faith, hope, and charity.

We tell clients that Mastered Eating involves:

1. letting go of relationships with an eating disorder. It's too busy thinking about itself, and therefore doesn't serve me any more
2. risking life while leaning into faith; trusting that you'll get through this moment because you got through every other moment you've experienced so far
3. understanding that mistakes and failures are data; they don't determine your value
4. practicing trust in your body, your recovery, and something greater than yourself
5. letting go of false beliefs that the culture, other people, and/or you have about your body
6. practicing internal stillness
7. reflection (self-study)
8. repeating all of the above.

As a former client says:

> For me, mastered eating involves letting go of rigidity, letting go of control, letting go of obsessive thoughts, and letting go of worry that one piece of food may forever impact my body or how others view me. Rather, food is energy for me. Period.

Our clients can master how to trust and care for their bodies and their recoveries. During Mastered Eating, clients integrate the truth that caretaking doesn't end with the body or the mind. Recovery teaches clients ways to care for the spiritual body or core self. These skills strengthen self-care "muscles" through daily practices including:

- rigorous honesty
- prayer
- setting intentions
- gratitude
- spiritual adoration
- experiencing nature
- experiencing fellowship
- art, music, dance.

These practices come from places in the self that channel and amplify the spiritual: body, mind, and soul. Now, we invite them to expand their mastery to other facets of life. This requires commitment to being in:

- fit nutritional condition
- fit thinking condition
- fit emotional regulation condition
- fit spiritual condition.

These practices begin to reveal answers to "Who am I without and/or beyond my eating disorder?" One of my former patients is a yoga teacher. The other day, she told me:

> During my yoga training, I realized that if I was really practicing yoga, I could not continue to practice my eating disorder. A spiritual life and eating disorder cannot exist in the same body. That doesn't mean I never ever struggle or stop growing in my recovery. I do. But I remain committed to practicing rigorous honesty in my relationship with my authentic self and other people. My eating disorder has no place in that. It's hard to let go of my "someone with an eating disorder" identity. But I cannot hold the yogic identity and the eating disorder identity in the same space, in the same self. So I made a daily decision to choose yoga.

Her comments reflect the union (aka yoga) of living in and with purpose. Our purpose can be writing books, caring for children, caring for the elderly, caring for the sick, performing accounting, performing music, performing surgery, teaching, computing, driving, farming, building, being with our loved ones, broadcasting, managing, counseling, worshipping, skiing, fire-fighting, marriage, pregnancy, adoption, pet rescue, snow plowing, dredging, policing, lawyering, forest management, and countless other things.

When we are fully in our purpose, there is no room for the eating disorder.

Unplugging the Eating Disorder

Earlier in the book we said that recovery cuts into the energy of an eating disorder, and its influence on the person's life. Recovery frees the people in our care to explore and grow into who they are *without* disordered energy. Plus, recovery's transformative energy and skills seep blessedly into all parts of life.

Because the disorder's energy is strong and stubborn, clients must still practice plugging in their recovery energy—even during Mastered Eating.

I think of a colleague's client who mastered using their clear and assertive voice to articulate their food needs. Their eating statements are unplugged from eating disorder energy. They easily say things like:

- I need to eat now.
- Excuse me, server, does bread come with this entree?
- I think I'll have the small shake, even though the large shake is on special today.
- I got a small shake last time, but I'm in the mood for more today. What other sizes do you have?

However, the client reported that they don't yet feel at ease speaking directly about other nourishment they need.

CLIENT: I wish I could tell my boss I need a day off the way I tell my husband I need to stop and eat lunch on our weekend road trips.

RD: OK, well, what have you learned about speaking up about food?

CLIENT: I learned it's scary, and it was nerve-wracking the first few times I spoke up about it with my husband.

RD: How do you feel in those food conversations now?

CLIENT: Pretty calm, actually. He gets it and stuff like pulling off the highway to get lunch doesn't seem like a big deal to him.

RD: OK. Well, why did you keep practicing how to express your food needs to your husband, even though it was nerve-wracking at first?

CLIENT: Because I learned that my body and I come first. I'm no longer willing to feed my body only when it's convenient for someone else, or not eat when I'm afraid that it might inconvenience someone else.

RD: Let's talk about that fear of inconveniencing someone else, because that's kind of a food fear.

CLIENT: There's not much to say, because no one *is* inconvenienced when I eat or speak up clearly. I get that now.

RD: OK. When it comes to your job, can you use any skills you learned about speaking up for food?

CLIENT: Yes, I already see that it's the same thing with work. I need to voice my needs for a day off. I need to come first in this situation too.

RD: Then, what's holding you back?

CLIENT: I don't have a disordered relationship with work like I had a disordered relationship with food! And, I'm afraid I'll get fired.

RD: Hmm.

CLIENT (CHUCKLING): Or, maybe I never considered that I might have a disordered relationship with work?

RD: Or maybe it's a "disordered" perception of what putting yourself first at work looks like? Your perspective is clearer with food because your eating disorder was wrecking your life. Work is more subtle. But do you see the common link between the two situations?

CLIENT (CHUCKLING): Kind of obvious, isn't it?

RD: Sure, but that doesn't mean it's easy. Finding responsible ways to put yourself first is part of taking good care of yourself. It's overall wellness. It's grist for you and your therapist!

CLIENT: Ugh, I have more work to do.

RD: True; there will always be more work to do when you're willing to grow.

In effect, this client is beginning to answer: "Who am I beyond my eating disorder?" It's dark and painful inside an eating disorder, but it seems safer and more predictable that what's outside. Truth be told, life beyond an eating disorder is far less predictable, and this presents spiritual challenges. We use analogies like the following to illustrate this aspect of recovered life.

Inside your house, you can predict a zero percent chance of rain today. On the TV this morning, a meteorologist predicted 80 percent chance of rain. Outside your house, it might rain and it might not. How is that possible? Because no one (not even a meteorologist) controls the weather. Prediction is not predetermination.

The weather is. Period. Full stop. We live in and with the weather. You might say that we have a relationship with weather, but it doesn't have a relationship with us. Unlike weather, we are sentient beings with will and the agency to act. No matter what the weather "does," we choose how to respond.

We can make absurd, self-defeating choices that create waves of harm to self and others:

- Deny weather's existence.
- Never leave the house (and live without food, wind, seeing a forest, etc.).
- Wear a swimsuit in a blizzard.
- Wear a parka and snow pants on 100-degree days.
- Stop in panic and paralysis when a tornado warning sounds.

We can also make smart, affirming, safe, and/or sound choices:

- Seize time on sunny says for a walk.
- Visit the Grand Canyon.
- Wear a raincoat in the rain, parka in the snow, wicking t-shirt in the desert.
- Go immediately to the basement during a tornado warning.
- Shovel snow so we can reach the car, bus, or subway.

Like the weather outside the protection of a house, life beyond the pseudo-protection of an eating disorder exists. Like everyone else, recovered people don't always like what happens in life and don't always respond wisely.

The Cultural Climate

Before, during, and after treatment and recovery, the people in our care walk through our cultural climate. To them (and many others) this climate often feels like daily downfalls of acid rain. Feel free to add dozens (or hundreds) more items to this short list:

1   Thousands of marketing messages assuring you that you are not [fill in the blank] enough as you are.
2   Thousands of marketing messages accusing you of failure if you ever feel uneasy—and insisting that you buy something to "fix" any discomfort.
3   If any of these "fixes" don't work, and/or make things worse, it's your fault. (See item 1.)
4   Outposts of the multibillion-dollar weight loss industry in every city and hamlet.
5   Aisles of foods labeled: health, lo-fat, no-fat, no-carb, hi-fiber, sugar-free, real sugar, gluten-free, dairy-free, GMO-free, grass-fed, cage-free, natural, real ingredients, and so on.

The culture often deems some well-balanced, nourishing foods "healthy." But that designation can change quickly.

Let's take chicken eggs for an example. Over the past few decades, chicken eggs were considered healthy for a while, until another (usually weight-loss) fad identified them as bad for our health.

The winds (and the "research") changed back and forth among unhealthy, not healthy enough, not healthy if you eat the yolk, not healthy if you eat the white, healthy again—perhaps after detouring through an "only duck (or platypus or dinosaur) eggs are healthy" phase.

Full disclosure: chicken eggs aren't changing. They still come from chickens and have all the essential amino acids we need. They don't have *all* the nutrition we need—even an egg can't be all things to all people.

What changes is cultural messages (most of them myths) about eggs—and many other foods.

People in recovery develop multiple methods to resist, respond to, and protect themselves from the acid rain:

- well-developed and calibrated BS detectors (aka, healthy skepticism) regarding attitudes, behaviors, myths, and marketing about food and bodies
- alternatives to screen time and other platforms that broadcast signals likely to overload BS detectors, sanity, and reality
- practices that keep them in tune with their inner wisdom, experience, and reality (see fit mental, emotional and spiritual condition above)
- patronizing yoga, dance, and fitness facilities without mirrors
- telling personal trainers, fitness instructors, yoga teachers, etc. not to weigh them, comment on their body, or give "food tips"
- using physicians and other healthcare providers who integrate health at every size (HAES), recovery-informed, and/or trauma-informed approaches.

Of course, other people also live in, and are influenced by, our cultural climate. Therefore, people in recovery must develop tools to deal with other people's attitudes, behaviors, and words about food and bodies.

One of our patients described the challenges of going to lunch with her friend one day:

> As we walked in the door, we heard people at a table nearby say: "So now that you're not running marathons any more, you're going to eat less, right? How much did you lose last week?" We sat down and the server eagerly explained the menu's entire paleo section. The next minute, my friend was complaining about the weight she gained while on vacation.
>
> At first, my biggest problem was having all those voices be someone else's, and not mine. I felt like an oddball left out of having someone else's weight issues affect me and being able to "get away with" choosing a "forbidden" diet meal. Then I felt a short urge to give in to my eating disorder symptoms.
>
> I'm happy to report how quickly the urge was replaced by knowing that those symptoms were scarier than the pastrami on pumpernickel I was ready to order. I felt satisfied and safe acting committed to my recovery; feeling how much more it means to me than these possible

pitfalls. I felt grateful for my recovery, which made it easier to accept that all this diet chatter was—well, that it just was. From there, it was a small step to say a short silent prayer for all of those folks, and me, too.

Many recovered people get involved in challenging and changing the culture, taking their share of responsibility for what Jewish tradition calls *tikkun olam*: repairing the world. But even world repairers must practice acceptance.

Every human faces the spiritual challenge of accepting life on life's terms. Each one of us responds imperfectly and, sometimes, creatively.

Experiencing New Knowledge

Earlier in this chapter, we discussed the neuroscience behind mastery "Eureka!" moments. Mastery moments bring "new" knowledge to our lives (including our challenges). Analogies help me explain mastery to clients. Here's one of them.

Imagine picking up a guitar for the first time. You need weeks of dedication, practice, and concentration to learn the most basic chords. You also need tolerance for frustration and pain (strings and frets hurt before fingers develop calluses).

With time and practice, your finger work, strumming, picking, and chord-reading competency grows. With more time and practice, you become aware enough to play chords without looking down at the instrument or at sheet music. Now, you can look at others while you sing. Pleasure and competence render pain tolerance irrelevant.

With even more time and practice, you memorize and learn to play and sing songs composed by other people. You integrate and embody hundreds of minutely executed movements to perform confidently. Perhaps you join a cover band, playing famous artists' music with joy and verve—whether you faithfully replicate an original recording or present your own interpretation.

Then one day (when mindlessly plucking strings while distracted by something else), a phrase of music suddenly pops or flows into your mind. You've never heard it before, but it's fully formed. Eureka! In that mastered moment, you composed a snippet of music.

In yoga, we learn that our work isn't complete when "shift happens" or we experience moments of flow. You'd be quickly bored if you play only that same phrase in the future. You need more snippets to build a song, a symphony, or an opus.

Mastering recovery and life demand that clients keep practicing skills and decisions aligned with recovery. Clients can explore all they want, while continuing to practice following inner wisdom and doing the next right thing.

Our clients gather fabulous (and transferable) skills while learning how to eat and to hear their inner wisdom. In recovery, they use their voice to ask for what they need. They create healthy and responsive boundaries with exercise, eating, partners, children, bosses, and more. They master much more than eating.

Experience provides evidence that ups and downs derail our clients' lives less frequently. Like guitar practice, recovery practice can generate new knowledge and flow.

For instance, people can (and do) re-perceive some characteristics of their previous disorder(s), and then transform them into mastery characteristics.

When veteran (and recovered) therapist and author Carolyn Costin had an eating disorder, she was also diagnosed with anxiety. She acknowledges retaining some characteristics of anxiety (intense energy) and compulsion (intense focus). However, Carolyn now considers—and uses—intense energy and focus as characteristics that channel life energy and help her be of service to others.

Notes for Nutritionists

Instead of goal-oriented structure and tool gathering, Mastered Eating nutrition sessions take on new dynamics. Storytelling replaces ritual food logging, troubleshooting replaces repetitive skill building, confident eating makes meal plans moot, and reflection drives the conversation.

We need fewer sessions—bi-monthly, monthly, or quarterly sessions, and/or some periodic wellness check-ins.

When we meet, clients do more of the talking and dietitians do more of the listening. They come back to us with reports, highlights, and observations. One mastered eater sat down and, like an author at a book reading, calmly shared her story:

> There I was at my sister's wedding in Utah. Her scrawny body in the white dress made me cringe. I didn't feel any envy. A few times, I thought of restricting or purging when watching her eating. Honestly, the thoughts were few, fleeting, and empty. As I was watching them, they seemed cartoonish. I didn't give into them because I already know that leads to things I don't want in my life. I was able to have the thoughts, process my feelings, and remain present. If anything, the wedding strengthened my commitment to my recovery. I felt a strong sense of pride for where I am now, compared to where I started.

We also troubleshoot alongside our clients:

> I have a long trip planned to Europe and want to start thinking about things that may come up. I know myself. I will want to try all the

yummy foods in Italy and Poland. But I don't want that to jeopardize my recovery. I don't want symptoms putting a dent into my trip. Can you help me strategize around this?

We act as co-explorers when they look for patterns in their current relationships, and how or whether those patterns reflect old, problem patterns. When symptoms or urges rear their head, they call us back into action. In turn we call them into action:

RD: I know something is up if you call me for a session before our monthly check-in. So, what's going on?

THEM: I want to do some thinking about what happened at the gala because I went in feeling prepared and confident. So, I'm utterly surprised that I considered purging there. Even though I didn't use symptoms it felt scary to get that close to them. I never want to go back. What do we do?

RD: How about looking at the events of the day and evening together?

THEM: Yeah; that would help me understand better my urge to purge?

RD: I agree. Let's get started.

While the sessions are less frequent and prescriptive, clients still need us as:

- role models for boundary-setting, balanced eating, self-care, etc.
- supportive coaches to acknowledge, validate, troubleshoot, and guide
- partners in navigating the big picture (find non-eating disorder identities, communities, and practices that resonate with recovery)
- partners in navigating the details (are there any meditation centers in the western suburbs?).

The Light in Me Bows to the Light in You

A person in the throes of an eating disorder can appear to be selfless. In reality, they often give away their energy, attention, and self because they do not feel worthy of them. Eating disorders fuel this dark, chaotic, and painful pattern. Ironically, eating disorders guide the person inward to deprivation, silence, and isolation. Instead of connecting to others and community, this kind of selflessness dims the authentic self.

I sometimes think we could rename recovery as uncovery. Through this long and winding journey, the people in our care lift the eating disorder lampshade covering an inner light they have by virtue of being alive. In this "new" light of uncovery/recovery, they glimpse what has always been: their authentic self.

A valuable gift of Mastered Eating is accepting—in body, mind, and soul—that there is finally enough. There is enough nutrition and light. Often, there is enough to share. We see recovered and recovering clients become metaphoric lamplighters. They don't brag about and proselytize for their light, or use it to measure their value. They use their light in the service of others and self. The lamplight has value in and of itself; no need for shade from expectation and judgment.

You can't measure authentic service in pounds per square foot, lumens, or other numerical values (spoiler alert: relationships ahead!). This kind of sharing service is selfless and, if you will, self*more*. It happens within, and in the service of, genuine relationships. Gratitude, compassion, and empathy manifest in selfless-and-selfmore service. Service lights our way into community and belonging. It unites people in communities which can, in turn, nourish their authentic, belonging members.

In short, we see recovered people willingly (and finally) care for themselves and for things greater than themselves.

> When I genuinely acknowledge the light in myself, I then see the light in others. I feel such gratitude in those moments. I feel every one of my cells saying "*namaste.*" The light within me bows to the light within you.

We see clients and former clients take pride in their mastery. This pride is different from old and futile attempts to overcompensate for fear. Rooted in gratitude for growth, clients welcome genuine pride and joy in mastery— without any need to broadcast it to the world. They certainly reserve the right to walk up to a stranger and shout: "I'm a warrior!" But they care more about what they've learned than what others think.

When clients leave the nutrition nest with mastery, others notice their purpose-filled energy. It radiates and invites others toward transformation. There is meaning far beyond their experience of the eating disorder, as this former client explains:

> I know that my body is healthy and happy. It works in better rhythm than it ever did before. My energy is incredible, and I feel at home in my body. My sleeping, eating, and menstruation are in sync. I know ways to self-soothe, self-nourish, and keep in balance—and I practice them. Willingly! Movement and exercise energize me, rather than depleting and obsessing me.

> Recently, a recovered friend and I were talking about our early days in treatment and what we wanted from recovery back then. I would've said that the *most* I could hope for was eating without throwing up. Or, eating with only half of my muscles clenched, instead of 100 percent.

I guess I didn't have the capacity to imagine what ended up happening. Eventually, instead of staying home in my room for Thanksgiving, I went with my family to my Grandma's. I ate with clenched muscles and just barely kept from purging. After a couple of years, I could tolerate the company and the dinner, but wish I was somewhere else. Eventually, I mostly felt calm at Thanksgiving, and saw that as proof that I was eating "normally."

Last November, I went over early to help Grandma *make* Thanksgiving dinner. We were rushing around the kitchen all playful and goofy. In the middle of all this, I stopped and realized I was feeling *joy!* Joy about feeling close to Grandma and sharing the love she puts into Thanksgiving. Joy about getting to see my cousins—so we could *eat* together!

I had goosebumps. Wow. My recovered life isn't barely tolerating food or taking deep breaths between each bite. It is living a life where food is one occasion for relishing and experiencing love in my family. This is my new normal. I never would have imagined. Wow, just wow.

We've witnessed recovered clients pursue helping careers in yoga, science, education, nursing, therapy, and even nutrition! Their purpose-filled living finally makes relationships with other people, places, and things more important than the disorder. Some leap into great unknowns like pregnancy. The common thread is simply breathing and living as a "human being, not a human doing."

We feel authentic awe when clients and former clients use their inherent power and mastery, knowing they are writing their own story. We see them use their "having been there" perspective to help other people learn how to transcend.

Mastered eaters integrate more of their inner wisdom and add new parts to their life. Their layers (or *koshas*) unite. Relationships flow. Life moves forward. This is mastery in action; yoga in action.

They feel new "superpowers" of joy, freedom, liberation, peace, acceptance, intimacy, and stability. Months and years of practice provide a spiritual "sense of smell" to sniff out and unplug eating disorder thoughts, voices, and behaviors before they create chaos. They know how to rise up and respond with poise and purpose.

Commencement

Ideally, our clients are integrating layers of life and self. Relationships flourish. Life keeps on life-ing. The people in our care practice self-study, acceptance, surrender while following their purpose.

Some folks leave our care. A few of them may send photos of their wedding day, kids, or pets. They may tell us when they divorce, lose a job, or became ill.

Other people in our care don't "leave" completely; they check in monthly or every few months. We willingly meet them where they are; note the changes, growth and, if needed, co-mentor them through challenges like divorce or illness.

"Finishing the work" is not a goal or expectation in therapy, psychiatry, medical care, and yoga therapy. However, eating disorders nutrition work has a fairly clear "finishing the work" line: the person knows how to eat. When a client is ready to leave the nutrition nest, it's time for a sacred acknowledgment that this body of work is over (at least for now).

Integrated Eating clinicians offer a "commencement" session to mark the occasion. Often, dietitian and client are ending a long relationship. They may have seen each other and exchanged conversation more frequently than with some members of their families. Like other commencements, these moments of goodbyes generate joy, sadness, and other contradictions (or paradoxes).

We honor the work the client has done and continues to do. We say: "I know you have the skills and practice to make recovery a priority. I am honored to work with you."

Sometimes a client will respond with statements like: "You saved my life!" or "It's all your doing" or "I could not have done this without you."

We reply with words like these:

- I appreciate that you feel this way. In truth, you saved yourself. This has been a co-creation, even when you felt like we were on opposite teams.
- Other members of our treatment team and I advocated for your body when your eating disorder made it hard to advocate for yourself. It took courage to stay with us.
- You know how to eat. You have practiced the structure. Your senses are attuned so you know what's going on inside and outside of you and so you can be in connection with the food you eat.
- Together we helped *you* navigate your recovery. Now you're a mastered eater and finding mastery in your life.
- You are still pushing into unknown challenges, questions, and obstacles. I know that you know how to practice faith and courage when afraid. You know how to listen to your gut and let your inner wisdom guide you onward.
- You have precious tools now, including self-care, self-acceptance, self-compassion, self-surrender, and self-love.
- You emerge a warrior, willing and ready to be of service to your self and to things greater than your self.
- I'm here and my door is always open. I believe you'll know if you ever need support from me or anyone else on your treatment team. Thank you for receiving our help and know that we are grateful for all you taught us.
- We are honored to walk beside you as guides and witnesses.

Usually, these "commencements" wrap up with hugs all around, a few tears, and reflections.

Eating disorders recovery work demands a lot from the patient, their family, their treatment team, and others. Not everyone heals. The work is still awe-inspiring.

For dietitians, the awe flows from recognizing how our work stimulates much more than nutrition education. We witness how science, dietetics, and yoga feed malnourished bodies, minds, and spirits. And, we witness how patients nourish us. These are awesome people.

While they may gush with gratitude for our guidance, they teach, too. May we strive toward gratitude for all we learn from the people in our care.

Namaste.

Bibliography

Barrett, M., Hardman, R., and Richards, P.S. The role of spirituality in eating disorder treatment and recovery. In M. Maine, B. Hartman McGilley, and D. Bunnell (Eds.), *Treatment of Eating Disorders: Bridging the Research-practice Gap* (London, UK: Academic Press, 2010). pp. 367–386.

Csikszentmihalyi, M. *Flow: The Psychology of Optimal Experience* (New York: HarperCollins, 1991).

Lee, J.J.K. *Receiving God's Deeper Messages: The Pilgrimage of a Truth-Seeking Christian* (Bloomington, Ind: iUniverse, 2005). Merton quote. p. 26.

Rogers, C. *On Becoming A Person: A Therapist's View of Psychotherapy* (Boston: Houghton Mifflin, 1961).

Index

For Product Safety Concerns and Information please contact our EU
representative GPSR@taylorandfrancis.com
Taylor & Francis Verlag GmbH, Kaufingerstraße 24, 80331 München, Germany